PREPARING FOR DISEASE X

LESSONS LEARNED FROM THE GENDERED IMPACTS OF THE COVID-19 PANDEMIC IN THE PACIFIC

NOVEMBER 2024

ASIAN DEVELOPMENT BANK

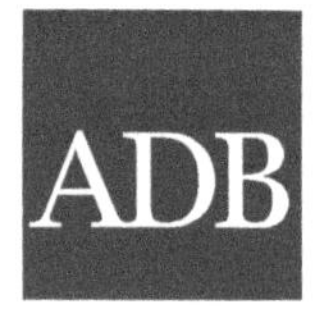

CONTENTS

FIGURES AND BOXES

ACKNOWLEDGMENTS

This report is based on work undertaken under Asian Development Bank (ADB) Technical Assistance (TA) 6549-REG: *Strengthening Gender Outcomes in Pacific COVID-19 Response and Recovery*. Overall, the regional TA project objective is to strengthen the institutional and technical capacity for progressing gender equality outcomes in Pacific developing member countries (DMCs), particularly in the context of response and recovery from the coronavirus disease (COVID-19). It supports Pacific DMCs to (i) identify gender mainstreaming opportunities and innovative and transformative gender projects and programs, (ii) strengthen DMC capacity to implement and monitor gender equality actions, and (iii) strengthen gender partnerships and knowledge among Pacific DMCs. The outcomes are directly linked to the ADB's Strategy 2030 (specifically, operational priority 2 on accelerating progress in gender equality) and Sustainable Development Goal 5 (achieve gender equality and empower all women and girls).

The preparation of *Preparing for Disease X: Lessons Learned from the Gendered Impacts of the COVID-19 Pandemic in the Pacific* benefited from the contributions and efforts of several individuals.

This report was written by Hannah Jay and Aleta Moriarty. The report was prepared under the generous guidance of Malika Shagazatova, senior social development specialist (Gender and Development), Gender Equality Division (CCGE), Climate Change and Sustainable Development Department (CCSD). Valuable recommendations were provided by Rachel Mary Anne Basas, gender officer; and Ingrid FitzGerald, former senior gender and social development officer assigned to the Pacific Liaison and Coordination Office, Pacific Department. Jan Andrew Orocay, gender knowledge management officer provided critical support in ensuring this publication's compliance with institutional guidelines; and Jaimie Lou Sarmiento and Ma. Celia Guzon, senior operations assistants, provided invaluable administrative assistance and coordination with relevant departments in ADB to make this publication a reality. Special thanks to Monina Gamboa, consultant, for providing editorial services. Much gratitude to Samantha Hung, director, CCGE, CCSD who provided indispensable guidance and support throughout the development of the report.

The manuscript underwent rigorous peer review by Keiko Nowacka, principal social development specialist (Gender and Development), as well as by experts in the health sector: Cebele Wong, health specialist, and Ki Fung Kelvin Lam, health specialist, both of the Human and Social Development Sector, Sectors Group.

We express our sincere appreciation to all these individuals for their expertise, dedication, and contributions to this work. Their collective efforts have significantly enriched the quality and depth of this publication.

ABBREVIATIONS

ADB	Asian Development Bank
AI	artificial intelligence
CEFM	child, early, and forced marriage
COVID-19	coronavirus disease
DMC	developing member country
FSM	Federated States of Micronesia
FWCC	Fiji Women's Crisis Centre
GBV	gender-based violence
GDP	gross domestic product
PNG	Papua New Guinea
PPE	personal protective equipment
RMI	Republic of the Marshall Islands
SRH	sexual and reproductive health
TA	technical assistance
UN	United Nations
UNDP	United Nations Development Programme
UNICEF	United Nations Children's Fund

EXECUTIVE SUMMARY

Coined by the World Health Organization, "Disease X" represents a hypothetical, future infectious disease of unknown etiology and origin and is considered a placeholder for an unforeseen pathogen, posing a public health risk. The unpredictability and potential danger of Disease X highlight the necessity for preparedness.

Research indicated there is a risk of experiencing a pandemic like the coronavirus disease (COVID-19) in one's lifetime, with a probability of about 38%. Given that over 7 million people died globally during the COVID-19 pandemic, preparedness for the next pandemic is critical.

A gender-inclusive response to Disease X can be shaped by what we have learned from COVID-19. The pandemic's gendered impacts in the Pacific provide vital insights for preparing for future pandemics and health emergencies. A gender-sensitive approach is crucial for effective and equitable pandemic response and recovery for the next pandemic that addresses the specific needs and challenges faced by women and girls.

The intended audience of this report primarily comprises policymakers and health and gender equality professionals in the Pacific region. It is especially relevant to those working in public health, economic development, food security, disaster preparedness, and gender equality portfolios. The report aims to inform these stakeholders by providing them with an exhaustive analysis of the gendered impacts of the COVID-19 pandemic to support and develop more equitable and effective policies and programs to ensure that future health crises do not exacerbate existing gender inequalities. The detailed recommendations are intended to be a resource for shaping policies and interventions that address the specific needs of women and marginalized groups, promoting a more inclusive approach to health in the Pacific in the event of future crises.

The Gendered Impacts of COVID-19 in the Pacific Region

The COVID-19 pandemic disproportionately affected women and girls in the Pacific region. This was evident in the predominantly female health sector. The interruption of medical supply chains and limited procurement during the pandemic endangered frontline women health care workers, with nurses in Papua New Guinea (PNG) organizing strikes over the lack of personal protective equipment (PPE) and inadequate public health measures.

There were equity issues in the uptake of vaccines. In some Pacific island countries, women were less likely than men to receive a COVID-19 vaccine, for a range of reasons, including lack of understanding on or access to the vaccine. In Kiribati, PNG, Samoa, Solomon Islands, and Tonga, women were less likely to receive the first two doses, particularly among older women and those in urban areas.

Women's access to COVID-19 information and prevention measures was impacted by gender gaps in literacy, education, and technology, limited internet access and the closure of women's spaces. In PNG, over 50% of women respondents reported being either unsure of or against accepting vaccines for COVID-19 due to a lack of information.

Women were economically impacted by border closures and travel restrictions: 77% of women-owned businesses reported a decline in revenue during the pandemic, compared to 65% of male-owned businesses. As the formal sector contracted, more women moved to informal work. Female-dominated export industries, such as fisheries and handicrafts, were heavily impacted, with large revenue and job losses. Border closures and supply chain issues impacted food security across the region. As supplies contracted, food prices increased, generating increased risks for women and girls.

Women's crisis centers and gender-based violence (GBV) service providers reported a surge of reports of gender-based and intimate partner violence during the pandemic. In Fiji, GBV service providers reported an increase in reported incidence during April 2020, as Fiji imposed a lockdown in response to the pandemic. The Fiji Women's Crisis Centre recorded the same number of incidents from February to April 2020 as they had for the whole of 2019.

Access to services and safe shelters for survivors was limited due to closures and reduced capacity, forcing some women to remain with their abusers. The provision of clinical care for sexual assault survivors faced challenges, although specific constraints and measures taken are not well-documented. Likewise, women's and girls' access to sexual and reproductive health (SRH) services was disrupted.

The COVID-19 pandemic had a profound impact on Pacific women, reversing progress toward gender equality and widening existing gender gaps. Women faced disproportionate economic challenges, with a marked decline in women-owned businesses and increased vulnerability in low-wage and informal sectors. Additionally, the burden of unpaid care work expanded for women, further limiting their economic opportunities. Reported incidences of GBV increased, while at the same time, specialist services faced operational barriers to service continuity. This regression in gender equality highlights the critical need to learn from the pandemic and implement targeted, gender-responsive policies in future crisis responses to Disease X to ensure equitable and inclusive recovery for all.

Recommendations

The report contains recommendations to prepare and respond equitably to future pandemics and health emergencies drawn from vital lessons from the COVID-19 pandemic. These will help future-proof and build responsiveness within governments to respond to crises from a gender perspective. These include:

(i)   Surveillance as the first critical step involves improving the collection and analysis of health data, which should be disaggregated by gender and disability status. The absence of such data during the COVID-19 pandemic posed challenges in understanding how different groups were affected and in tailoring health responses. This includes developing systems that can efficiently collect, integrate, and analyze data from diverse sources with a gender and disability lens.

(ii)   Preparedness involves ensuring that public health measures, such as plans for quarantine, travel restrictions, and public space closures, are informed by the increased gendered risks identified during the COVID-19 crisis, such as GBV. This also includes preparing health care facilities, particularly isolation units and intensive care facilities, with gender considerations in mind. Stockpiling essential medical supplies, including PPE, menstrual hygiene products, medications, and necessary equipment, is crucial, considering the heightened risks faced by women health workers during PPE shortages in the COVID-19 pandemic.

(iii) Improving response systems should include plans for the continuity of essential services such as education and SRH services, where disruptions disproportionately impacted women during the COVID-19 pandemic. Developing accessible continuity plans for these services is critical. Moreover, the response needs to involve consultation with women and girls, ensuring that recovery planning and preparedness measures are informed by their needs, particularly those from diverse backgrounds, including single parents, women with disabilities, and those living in rural areas.

(iv)   Last, responding and building resilience involves strengthening social protection systems to meet the needs of women and diverse gender groups more effectively. Stimulus packages need to be designed to reach women, including women-owned and -led micro, small, and medium-sized enterprises in the informal sector, ensuring income support and subsidies are gender-responsive, and promoting women's access to insurance for disasters and shocks.

Improving or putting in place care infrastructure to address the gender gap in unpaid household and care labor is crucial. This could include expanding accessible childcare systems, extending maternity and paternity leave provisions, ensuring more equitable distribution of household labor, and increasing support for elder care services.

Addressing the digital divide is also a key enabler for women and girls throughout the region. Internet access was critical for accessing COVID-19 information and pivoting businesses online during lockdowns, as well as supporting service delivery.

INTRODUCTION

The purpose of this report is to identify lessons learned and provide recommendations to prepare for Disease X based on an analysis of the gendered impacts of the coronavirus disease (COVID-19) on women and girls in the Pacific region.

The impact of the COVID-19 pandemic and measures taken to prevent the transmission of the disease exacerbated many existing gender inequalities in Pacific island countries and disproportionately affected women and girls.[1]

Research shows that there were impacts for women, including the increased risks of infection, increases in reported incidences of gender-based violence (GBV) and decreased access to clinical services, negative economic impacts, and potential long-term impacts on gender equality. Findings from the literature review on COVID-19 informed recommendations for preparedness efforts for Disease X or future pandemics and other health emergencies.

The methodology used to draw out recommendations for this report is based on a review and synthesis of available evidence on the impacts of the COVID-19 pandemic on gender equality across 14 countries in the Pacific during the pandemic health emergency from March 2020 to May 2023.

The review examined 228 resources, drawn from a systematic examination of secondary data from academic and bibliographic databases and gray literature published between the onset of the crisis in early 2020 and May 2023. The literature review was conducted using the following staged methodology:

Stage 1: Scan

A scan of a broad range of existing evidence on the impacts of COVID-19 on gender equality in Pacific island countries.

(i) **A keyword search** using terms such as "COVID-19," "pandemic," and "gender," and all the different countries in Google, Google Scholar, as well as bibliographic databases, starting with any systematic or comprehensive reviews.

---

[1] This report examines evidence from 14 Pacific island countries: the Cook Islands, Fiji, Kiribati, the Marshall Islands, the Federated States of Micronesia, Nauru, Niue, Palau, Papua New Guinea, Samoa, Solomon Islands, Tonga, Tuvalu, and Vanuatu. See Box 1 for introduction to Disease X.

(ii) **Using the snowball method**, additional sources and resources were identified that were cited within or otherwise referenced in the initial scan of documents, including sources referenced in documents outside of the inclusion criteria. Keywords included "gender," "COVID-19," "women," "men," "pandemic," "COVID," and Pacific island country names.

(iii) **Manual searches** were conducted to identify any additional studies or databases not available through the methods above.

(iv) **Networks** in the region were engaged to identify any additional sources such as women's networks, the Pacific Islands Forum, and multilateral agencies.

Stage 2: Evidence Mapping

All published evidence found in the scan were tracked and evaluated.

(i) **Track and map the evidence.** Details of each document were tracked, the relevant evidence contained within the document and details on the quality of the evidence, such as methodology of the study, sampling methodology if relevant, and the limitations of the evidence collected.

(ii) **Evaluate and screen the evidence.** Following the initial evidence scan, the evidence was screened and any duplicate studies or studies that do not meet the inclusion criteria were removed.

Stage 3: Analyze and Summarize the Evidence

Summarize the evidence. The evidence that met inclusion criteria was then coded, analyzed, and summarized for this report, drawing from pre-pandemic information to show any increase or decrease from baseline figures.

Limitations

This study had the following limitations:

(i) Countries in the literature were unevenly represented, with limited information available for smaller island states and countries in the North Pacific.

(ii) The impacts of the pandemic throughout its phases were difficult to examine due to the lack of longitudinal data.

(iii) Sex-disaggregated data on COVID-19 infection rates, hospitalizations, and vaccinations were limited across Pacific island countries.

(iv)   Limited evidence existed on the impact of the pandemic on girls, particularly young and adolescent girls, as well as on child sexual abuse disaggregated by sex.

(v)   The transition to online and remote gender-based violence (GBV) service delivery and its impact on accessibility was poorly documented.

(vi)   Information on the continuity of GBV prevention work and the impact of economic abuse was lacking.

(vii)   Limited evidence existed on the impact of the pandemic on child, early, and forced marriage (CEFM), as well as on unsafe abortion rates.

(viii)   There was a lack of independent evaluations on the effectiveness of government and development partner responses to the pandemic.

(ix)   There were limited disaggregated data on intersectional vulnerabilities and impacts. These gaps in data and evidence constrained the development of a full picture of impacts but emphasized the need for improvements in these areas in preparedness planning.

Box 1: Introduction to Disease X

"Disease X" refers to an unknown hypothetical pathogen that the World Health Organization (WHO) anticipates could lead to a major international epidemic.[a] This term serves as a placeholder for the next pandemic or health emergency, guiding global research and preparedness efforts for future pandemics.

M. Marani et al. state that due to environmental changes causing higher rates of disease transmission from animal hosts, the likelihood of experiencing pandemics similar to the coronavirus disease (COVID-19) is expected to increase significantly, potentially doubling in the next few decades.[b] The likelihood of experiencing a pandemic like COVID-19 in one's lifetime is about 38%.[c] Given that over 7 million people died globally during the COVID-19 pandemic and economic impacts were experienced globally, preparedness for the next pandemic is critical.[d]

[a]   WHO. 2022. *WHO to Identify Pathogens that Could Cause Future Outbreaks and Pandemics*. 21 November.
[b]   M. Marani et al. 2021. Intensity and Frequency of Extreme Novel Epidemics. *Proceedings of the National Academy of Sciences*. 118(35). e2105482118.
[c]   Gender in Humanitarian Action and Gender Based Violence Area of Responsibility. 2021.Gender and COVID-19 Vaccines: Listening to Women-Focused Organizations in Asia and the Pacific.
[d]   WHO. 2023. Director-General's opening remarks at the media briefing. 5 May.
Source: Authors.

THE SOCIOECONOMIC IMPACT OF THE COVID-19 PANDEMIC ON WOMEN AND GIRLS

The COVID-19 pandemic resulted in an unprecedented socioeconomic crisis with macroeconomic impacts on the Pacific region that disproportionately affected women. During this period, the region registered its worst economic performance in decades.[2] The impact on the economies of Pacific island countries was more severe than on any other region, with a 4.4% combined contraction in gross domestic product (GDP) between 2019 and 2021.[3] Tourism-dependent countries experienced a particularly sharp drop, with Fiji, Palau, and Samoa all suffering a 10% reduction in GDP as a result of restrictions put in place to curb the pandemic.

Across the region, women-owned businesses were significantly impacted by the pandemic. The Pacific Trade Invests (PTI) surveys showed that 77% of women-owned businesses in the Pacific experienced a decline in revenue during the pandemic, compared to 65% of male-owned businesses.[4] A government assessment in Tuvalu conducted in 2020 found similar results: 63% of women business owners reported their businesses were impacted by border closures, compared to 37% of men business owners. Income-generating activities dependent on tourism and handicraft sales (mostly led by women) were most affected, while businesses dominated by men, such as motorbike rentals, were largely unaffected.[5]

Gendered barriers in accessing financial support worsened the impact of COVID-19 for women entrepreneurs. The PTI business monitor reported in November 2021 that half of female-led or -owned businesses required financial support, compared to just 37% of male-led or -owned businesses. The report also showed that this gap had increased over time as the pandemic progressed.[6] Furthermore, a United Nations Economic and Social Commission for Asia and the Pacific (ESCAP) report found that women in Samoa accessed lower levels of finance during the COVID-19 pandemic, and small and medium enterprises led and/or owned by women overall experienced higher levels of financial vulnerability. The burden of increased unpaid care and household labor, as well as collateral shortfall and lower access to information and communication technology and business networks were particular barriers facing women.[7]

2   ESCAP. 2021. *Economic and Social Survey of Asia and the Pacific 2021: Towards Post-COVID-19 Resilient Economies*.

3   International Monetary Fund. 2022. Real GDP Growth. Quoted in S. Howes and H. Liu. 2022. The Pacific: Emerging from COVID, Slowly. DevPolicy Blog. 19 October.

4   PTI. 2021. Business Monitor Surveys. Quoted in Social Development Direct. 2022. *Women's Economic Empowerment in the Pacific. A Literature Review*. ADB.

5   Tuvalu Ministry of Health, Social Welfare and Gender Affairs. 2020. *Rapid Assessment of Socio-Economic Impacts of the Global COVID-19 Pandemic*.

6   PTI. 2021. *Pacific Business Monitor 2021: Female-Led/Female-Owned Focus*.

7   ESCAP. 2020. *Micro, Small and Medium-Sized Enterprises' Access to Finance in Samoa: COVID-19 Supplementary Report and Recommendations*.

Border closures and travel restrictions impacted women's businesses and their work. The Pacific tourism industry was significantly affected by widespread border closures. The sector, which accounted for around half of exports in countries such as Fiji, Samoa, and Vanuatu, suffered job losses.[8] In Fiji, women made up one-third of the tourism industry workforce, predominantly holding minimum wage positions, such as cleaners, restaurant staff, and receptionists, while a quarter held roles in management and professional capacities. Women were also extensively engaged in tourism-related businesses, such as floriculture, local food production, jewelry crafting, handicrafts, organic cosmetics, as well as spa and massage services.[9] In Tuvalu, women's handicraft groups lost their sources of income when international flights were canceled in early 2020 (footnote 5).

Women working in export industries, such as the tuna processing sector in Solomon Islands and the handicraft industries in Tonga and Samoa, were heavily impacted by COVID-19. There were reports of job losses in the tuna industry in Solomon Islands, with the combined impact of the COVID-19 pandemic and Tropical Cyclone Harold leading to the downsizing of the workforce, two-thirds of whom were women.[10] In a study looking at food systems in 2020, interviewees spoke of the economic impact of lockdowns and border closures on rural women's weaving opportunities. As one informant noted, "Most weaving comes from women, done in a group—however, because of the social isolation, women cannot come together and weave, so household income is declining. The baskets produced by women's weaving activities are often bought by diaspora communities in New Zealand and Australia, who may be facing their own unemployment pressures due to the COVID-19 crisis."[11]

Border closures and supply chain issues impacted food security across the region. As supplies contracted, food prices increased, generating increased risks for women and girls. Concerns around food insecurity were particularly prominent in the North Pacific, which is heavily reliant on imported foods. These challenges, coupled with efforts to manage shortages, panic buying, and domestic constraints, added further burdens on women and girls who were tasked with acquiring and preparing food.[12] A survey found that in Samoa, Solomon Islands, and Tonga,[13] more women faced difficulties in accessing an adequate amount of food compared to men.[14] In some countries in the Pacific, food insecurity was exacerbated by multiple overlapping crises, such as Tropical Cyclone Harold, which damaged crops across Solomon Islands and Vanuatu.[15]

Women across the Pacific shouldered additional unpaid care and household labor due to school closures and other impacts of the COVID-19 pandemic. Evidence available for some Pacific island countries shows that the impact of the pandemic increased the demands of care labor for women. There was some evidence on the detrimental impact of this increased burden on women's economic

---

[8]   E. Cliffe. 2020. *Feminist Future for the Pacific. White Paper for the Centre for Humanitarian Leadership*. Centre for Humanitarian Leadership.

[9]   Adventist Development and Relief Agency (ADRA), CARE, and Save the Children. 2021. *Fiji Gender, Disability and Inclusion Analysis COVID-19, TC Yasa, TC Ana*.

[10]   Cooperative for Assistance and Relief Everywhere (CARE). 2020. *Solomon Islands Gender, Disability and Inclusion Analysis for COVID-19 and Tropical Cyclone Harold*.

[11]   Australian Centre for International Agricultural Research. 2020.

[12]   Pacific Women Shaping Pacific Development. 2020. *GBV Situational Report*.

[13]   It found the opposite was true in Kiribati and Papua New Guinea (PNG).

[14]   Asian Development Bank (ADB) and UN Women. 2022. *Two Years On: The Lingering Gender Effects of COVID-19 in Asia and the Pacific*.

[15]   D. J. Steenbergen et al. 2020. COVID-19 Restrictions Amidst Cyclones and Volcanoes: A Rapid Assessment of Early Impacts on Livelihoods and Food Security in Coastal Communities in Vanuatu. *Marine Policy*, 121.

empowerment, but less on impacts on other areas of women's lives, such as continuing education, mental health, and time poverty. Women in various countries continued to carry out domestic tasks such as cooking, cleaning, and buying necessities and daily needs (Figure 1). Activities that are less time-consuming, such as decorating, making repairs, and managing bills, were shared more equally between women and men. Data from five countries showed that 13% of women and 10% of men spent increased time feeding, cleaning, and providing medical care for children (Figure 2). Importantly, this 13% figure does not include time spent supervising children's education. In Fiji, Solomon Islands, Tuvalu, and Vanuatu, women's unpaid labor increased due to caring for relatives migrating or returning from urban areas (footnote 14).

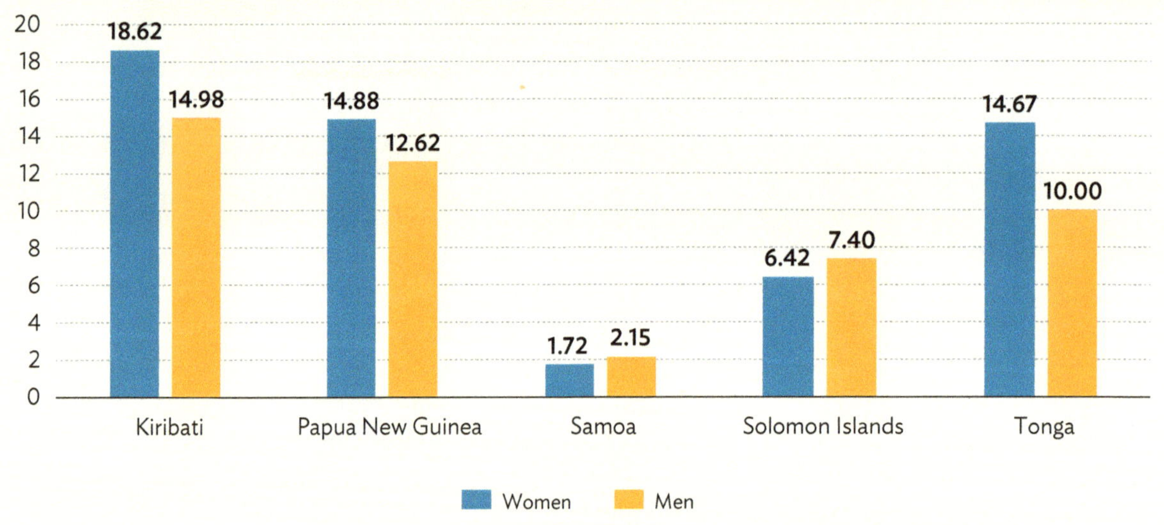

Figure 1: Proportion of People Who Noted Increased Time Spent on Doing Laundry and Cleaning Since the Onset of COVID-19, by Sex
(%; n = 11,845)

Notes: For women and men in Samoa, estimates for increases in time allocation on cleaning and doing laundry should be interpreted with caution as the number of respondents that chose this response category is less than 25. Respondents who reported "I don't know" or refused to respond were excluded from the analysis.
Source: Asian Development Bank and UN Women. 2022. *Two Years On: The Lingering Gendered Effects of the COVID-19 Pandemic in Asia and the Pacific.*

COVID-19 affected the division of household responsibilities, with a greater impact on women compared to men. In Kiribati, women reported spending 8% more time on domestic tasks compared to men, while in Papua New Guinea (PNG), the difference was slightly lower at 7.4% (footnote 14). Samoa showed a disparity with women spending approximately 66.7% more time than men, although this figure should be approached with caution due to the small number of respondents. Both Solomon Islands and Tonga displayed a 28.6% higher time investment by women in these domestic activities, indicating a substantial gender-based difference in the division of labor for household tasks during the pandemic period (footnote 14).

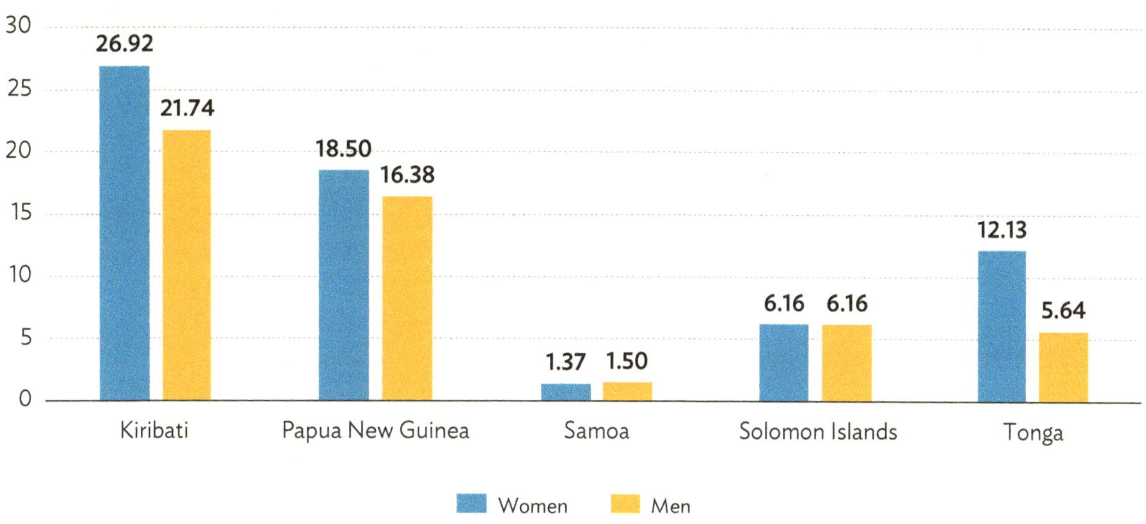

Figure 2: Proportion of People Who Noted Increased Time Spent on Feeding, Providing, Washing, Physical, and Medical Care for Children Since the Onset of COVID-19, by Sex
(%; n = 11,845)

Notes: For women and men in Samoa, estimates for increases in time allocation on cleaning and doing laundry should be interpreted with caution as the number of respondents that chose this response category is less than 25. Respondents who reported "I don't know" or refused to respond were excluded from the analysis.
Source: Asian Development Bank and UN Women. 2022. *Two Years On: The Lingering Gendered Effects of the COVID-19 Pandemic in Asia and the Pacific.*

According to available data, there is an increased load of extra unpaid household and caregiving duties placed on girls across the region. A survey conducted by Pacific Women Shaping Pacific Development, involving 21 adolescent girls aged 14–19 from various Pacific nations, revealed that these girls' responsibilities for caregiving at home have intensified.[16] The survey discovered that adolescent girls frequently took on the responsibilities of caring for siblings and children in the community, particularly when schools were closed, along with additional household chores. This role stems from traditional expectations for girls to assist their mothers and female relatives, who typically handle the majority of unpaid domestic work and childcare (footnote 14). Apart from this survey and study covering the broader region,[17] there was minimal detailed information available about how the pandemic affected unpaid caregiving and household labor when broken down by age group.

Despite the evidence showing an increased burden of labor for women, there have been few interventions in the region targeting the impact of additional care work on women and girls. Interventions that have been implemented are substantially limited in scale. For example, the Cook Islands provided support to families during the school closure in the form of one-off cash payments through the existing social protection system, and Samoa introduced special leave with pay for employees who needed to care for family members with suspected or confirmed COVID-19 infection.[18]

---

16   Pacific Women Shaping Pacific Development. 2020. *Thematic Brief: Impacts of the COVID-19 Pandemic on Adolescent Girls in the Pacific.*

17   Australian Centre for International Agricultural Research. 2023. *COVID-19 in the Indo-Pacific: Gendered Risks, Impact and Response.*

18   See Box 2 for the Cook Islands Social Protection system; UNDP. *COVID-19 Global Gender Response Tracker* (accessed 1 March 2022).

State of emergency orders and lockdowns associated with COVID-19 led to the closure of public transport or limiting of services in several Pacific island countries. Half of the population in PNG was impacted by disruptions to public transportation, as well as 33% of the population in Kiribati and 30% in Solomon Islands (footnote 14). While there were limited reliable data on the representation of women using public transport during the pandemic, a study conducted in PNG before the pandemic indicated that, in general, a higher proportion of women used public transportation compared to men.[19] Global information shows that safe and accessible public transport is crucial for women's mobility, facilitating access to employment and education and impacting women's time poverty.[20] Data from 2022 showed that public transport usage in Fiji had not recovered to pre-pandemic levels.[21]

Despite early concerns about disruptions to remittances, the projected decline in revenue was largely avoided and many countries in the Pacific experienced an increase in remittance inflows throughout the pandemic. In the early phase of the pandemic, there were concerns about the impact of a reduction in remittances, given these contribute such a large portion of GDP in many Pacific island countries.[22] There was particular concern in Tonga, which was among the highest receivers of remittances in the world in 2019, with remittance inflows comprising 38.5% of its GDP.[23] The majority of households in Tonga received some remittances and they were particularly important to the 22% of households that are female-headed.[24] Accounting for seasonal fluctuations, there was a documented initial drop in remittances in some countries; however, by 2022, remittance flows had either increased or stabilized.[25]

Social Protection

The COVID-19 pandemic exacerbated underlying socioeconomic conditions, including economic insecurity, poverty, inequality, and widespread informal employment. The crisis laid bare disparities and deficiencies in formal social protection systems regionally, revealing the vulnerability of many people, particularly women, who lacked sufficient protection against the pandemic's socioeconomic repercussions. As a result, many turned to traditional safety nets, which helped act as a buffer in this vacuum.

There was an increase in social protection investment in response to the COVID-19 pandemic. This partly reflected inadequate social protection before the crisis.[26] Countries that had preexisting social protection schemes were better able to respond quickly and distribute payments through existing mechanisms.

---

[19]   UN Women. 2014. *Ensuring Safe Public Transport with and For Women and Girls in Port Moresby*.

[20]   International Transport Forum. 2021. *COVID-19 Transport Brief; Gender Equality, The Pandemic, and a Transport Rethink*.

[21]   Google. 2022. *COVID-19 Community Mobility Report Fiji*.

[22]   Organisation for Economic Co-operation and Development. 2021. *COVID-19 Pandemic: Towards a Blue Recovery in Small Island Developing States*.

[23]   Global Knowledge Partnership on Migration and Development (KNOMAD). 2019. *Migration and Remittance Data Update: Remittances to low- and middle-income countries on track to reach $551 billion in 2019 and $597 billion by 2021*. World Bank.

[24]   UN Women. 2021. *Gender Equality Brief for Tonga*.

[25]   ADB Pacific Economic Monitor. 2022. *The Future of Social Protection in the Pacific*.

[26]   ADB Pacific Economic Monitor. 2020. *Preparing for Recovery*.

Gender-responsive measures were implemented in some Pacific island countries. Some schemes were specifically designed to address the gendered impacts of the COVID-19 pandemic. For example, the Cook Islands waived maternal health fees for recent migrants and those not already eligible for free government care and provided payments to families to offset the impacts of school closures (footnote 18). The Federated States of Micronesia (FSM) provided temporary waivers for medical expenses not covered by existing programs, and electricity subsidies to low-income households, including female-headed households.[27] However, these measures were limited in scope and were implemented for a restricted period.

Completion reports for Asian Development Bank (ADB)-financed COVID-19 response projects provide some information on the gendered access to social protection payments in Palau and the FSM. In Palau, women comprised 40.1% (1,934 recipients) of recipients of unemployment payments between May 2020–January 2021.[28] In the FSM, female-headed households comprised 34% of recipients of one-off payments made between December 2020 and September 2021 to 9,325 beneficiaries.[29] Self-reported data from UN Women showed more men accessing social protection grants in Samoa, Solomon Islands, and PNG, and more women accessing them in Kiribati and Tonga (footnote 14). The Pacific Islands Forum Secretariat noted that, in some Pacific island countries, the government reached the informal economy (where most women entrepreneurs are located) through one-off payments. However, the amounts were often too low to meet their needs.[30] For example, in Fiji, registered street hawkers were entitled to a Fiji dollars one-off government relief payment.[31] Likewise, fees were waived for market vendors, mostly women, in Fiji during 2020.[32]

Many of the social protection initiatives during the pandemic lacked sex-disaggregated data. While some inferences may be drawn from pre-pandemic sex-disaggregated data on access to social protection, this excludes those who were economically impacted by the pandemic and may have been eligible for social protection payments and support.[33] This reiterates the importance of not just ensuring such schemes reach women, but that effective data, disaggregated by gender, age, and disability status are collected.

Social protection coverage was patchy, and many vulnerable people were unable to access formal schemes, including many in the informal economy, i.e., people with disabilities, and those from the lesbian, gay, bisexual, transgender, intersex, queer plus community. People of diverse sexual orientation, gender identity, expression, and sex characteristics in Fiji faced barriers to government social protection programs due to a lack of information, stigma, and restrictive eligibility criteria for households based on normative family structures.[34]

---

[27] FSM Information Services. 2020. *President Panuelo Develops & Expands $14,000,000 of COVID-19 Related Social Protection Programming, Funded in Part by Asian Development Bank; Stranded Citizens to Receive an Additional $1,000 Per Person or $1,500 Per Family Application*. Press release. 15 December.

[28] ADB. 2022. *Palau : Health Expenditure and Livelihoods Support Program: Program Completion Report*.

[29] ADB. 2022. *Micronesia, Federated States of: Health Expenditure and Livelihoods Support Program*.

[30] Pacific Islands Forum Secretariat. 2020. *Forum Economic Ministers Meeting: Information Paper No. 4: Economic Empowerment of Women*.

[31] KPMG. 2020. *Fiji – Measures in Response to COVID-19*.

[32] R. Nasiko. 2023. Union Welcomes Reinstatement of Market Fees. *The Fiji Times*. 1 August.

[33] Fiji Women's Rights Movement. 2019. *Social Protection Schemes in Fiji*.

[34] Australian Aid/Edge Effect. 2021. *We Don't Do a Lot for Them Specifically: A Scoping Report on Gaps and Opportunities for Improving Diverse SOGIESC Inclusion in Cash Transfer and Social Protection Programs During the COVID-19 Crisis and Beyond*.

Confronted by a lack of formal social protection coverage, many people, particularly women, turned to subsistence agriculture and traditional community support, which acted as an informal safety net. Research across seven countries revealed that rural communities in the Pacific islands, which preserved traditional methods of food production, experienced greater resilience against the early effects of COVID-19.[35] The role of these traditional systems cannot be overemphasized as they have repeatedly provided a safety net for Pacific island citizens against economic shocks.[36]

Women's long-term financial stability was impacted by the drawing down of savings and retirement funds as a coping mechanism for the impacts of the COVID-19 pandemic on business and household finances. A rise in unemployment during the COVID-19 pandemic forced many in the region to access retirement funds to cover daily expenses. This policy was actively promoted across many countries in the region (footnote 25). Pre-pandemic information showed that women had less in retirement accounts than men, so while withdrawals impacted adversely on both men and women, due to already lower balances, women's finances were more substantially impacted.[37] This will likely impact women's economic security in the future, with limited access to alternative pension schemes available across the region.

Pacific countries are currently at a crucial juncture in determining the future of their social protection systems to enhance resilience against Disease X. The pandemic has highlighted the urgent requirement to invest in social protection, but many nations are constrained financially due to substantial expenditures incurred during the crisis. In Asia and the Pacific, the projected cost of establishing a social protection floor is highest for Pacific countries, averaging 6.5% of GDP in 2024 and expected to rise to 9.02% of GDP by 2030.[38] Utilizing the opportunities created by the pandemic, countries can build upon their emergency measures to strengthen their protection systems, aiming for universality, comprehensiveness, adequacy, and sustainability, including a robust social protection floor for all. At the same time, investing in traditional systems and agricultural development is likely to build resilience against exogenous shocks.

Nations that had invested in social protection systems before the onset of the COVID-19 crisis were better equipped to handle the pandemic's impact. This was evident in the cases of the Cook Islands, Fiji, Kiribati, Samoa, and Tonga, which efficiently utilized their preexisting social welfare structures and economic bases.[39] They swiftly implemented measures, such as temporary additional support for older people, individuals with disabilities, and children who were already beneficiaries of existing welfare programs (footnote 39).

---

35   C. E. Ferguson et al. 2022. *Local Practices and Production Confer Resilience to Rural Pacific Food Systems During the COVID-19 Pandemic*. *Marine Policy*, 137.

36   S. Feeny. n.d. *The Impact of the Global Economic Crisis on the Pacific Region*. Oxfam.

37   Pacific Private Sector Development Initiative (PSDI). 2022. *A Secure Retirement: Levelling the Playing Field for Women in the Pacific*.

38   M. Van der Auwera, A. van de Meerendonk, and A. R. Kumar. 2021. COVID-19 and Social Protection in Asia and the Pacific: Projected Costs for 2020–2030. *ADB Sustainable Development Working Paper Series*, No. 80. ADB.

39   C. Knox-Vydmanov and S. Satriana. 2022. *Social Protection in the Pacific and Timor-Leste: The State of Play*.

**Box 2: The Cook Islands Social Protection System
During the COVID-19 Pandemic**

The Cook Islands has one of the region's leading social protection systems. It is enshrined in its 1965 Constitution and guided by various legislation and strategies, such as the 1989 Welfare Act and the 2014 Welfare Amendment Act. The country's social protection system aims to safeguard vulnerable members of society and is driven by the Ministry of Internal Affairs and the Cook Islands National Superannuation Fund.

Prior to the pandemic, government spending on social protection was substantial, amounting to NZ$20.8 million in the fiscal year 2018, representing 4.0% of gross domestic product (GDP). Most of this expenditure was allocated to social assistance, specifically focusing on the old age allowance.

During the pandemic, the Cook Islands raised its social protection spending to NZ$23.6 million, equivalent to 5.5% of GDP, as part of its crisis response. This increase constituted a large portion of the government's operational budget and encompassed a comprehensive Economic Response Plan featuring various initiatives. These included a wage subsidy, training support, "Fees Free" program, exemptions from maternal health fees, unemployment and school closure benefits, an electricity discount, an emergency hardship fund, and one-time payments to individuals severely affected by job losses resulting from border closures. Benefiting from the existing social protection infrastructure, the government was able to swiftly implement these measures, helping to alleviate the pandemic's socioeconomic impacts.

The Cook Islands' initiatives in social protection mirror larger issues and patterns in the Pacific region. Traditional social safety nets in the Pacific are encountering strain due to urbanization, food insecurity, and migration, while formal systems remain relatively undeveloped.

There is a need to strengthen social safety nets in other countries, and build resilience against future shocks from climate change, disasters, and health emergencies. Despite the socioeconomic challenges posed by the pandemic, these efforts are crucial for sustaining social protection in the new normal.

Source: ADB. 2022. *Pacific Economic Monitor.*

THE GENDER DIMENSIONS OF THE ECONOMIC STIMULUS

During the crisis, all Pacific governments received economic stimulus packages to support COVID-19 efforts. The stimulus packages were designed to support those industries and sectors hardest hit by the crisis. The cost of stimulus across Fiji, PNG, Samoa, Vanuatu, Solomon Islands, and Tonga averaged 5.7% of GDP, ranging from 3.1% to 9% of GDP.[40]

While the stimulus per capita worked out as high as $547 in countries like Fiji, the impact of the stimulus was not gender-neutral (footnote 40). Social protection expenditures were less likely to reach women who predominantly operated in the informal sector, and many investments, such as those targeting infrastructure in Solomon Islands, were more likely to benefit male workers than investments in social infrastructure.

In many countries, the lack of gender-disaggregated data obscured the differential impacts of these stimulus packages on men and women. Without this data, it was challenging to design and implement policies that adequately address the unique needs and circumstances of women and to also assess the effectiveness of the packages themselves.

The ADB COVID-19 Pandemic Response Program was able to work with governments to leverage stimulus to deliver better outcomes for women.[41] In the Republic of the Marshall Islands (RMI), the health and economic stimulus package prioritized initiatives aimed at women and girls. These efforts encompassed extensive training in infection prevention and control for health workers, where 54% were women; economic assistance provided to business owners, with over a third being women; the distribution of water, sanitation, and hygiene and dignity kits to women and girls in households facing vulnerability; and the establishment of a GBV hotline with support services. These highlight, with appropriate targeting, how stimulus packages are a very powerful tool to drive gender equality outcomes.

While the stimulus was necessary and was pivotal in avoiding financial instability in the region,[42] the long-term impacts are still playing out (footnote 40). A significant level of inflationary pressure resulting from a variety of complex factors, including stimulus measures,[43] likely had a disproportionate impact on women across the Pacific. Inflation (Figure 3) tends to affect those with lower incomes

---

40   S. Howes and S. Surandiran. 2021. *Pacific COVID Economic Database*. Australian National University. Averages across the spreadsheet (accessed 14 August 2024).

41   ADB. 2022. *Health Expenditure and Livelihoods Support Program: Report and Recommendation of the President*. Project Number: 54358-001; Grant Number: 0766.

42   K. Wilkins. 2023. *Economic Developments in the South Pacific*. Reserve Bank of Australia.

43   D. Jef. 2023. *Recent Inflation Experiences in Asia and the Pacific*. International Monetary Fund.

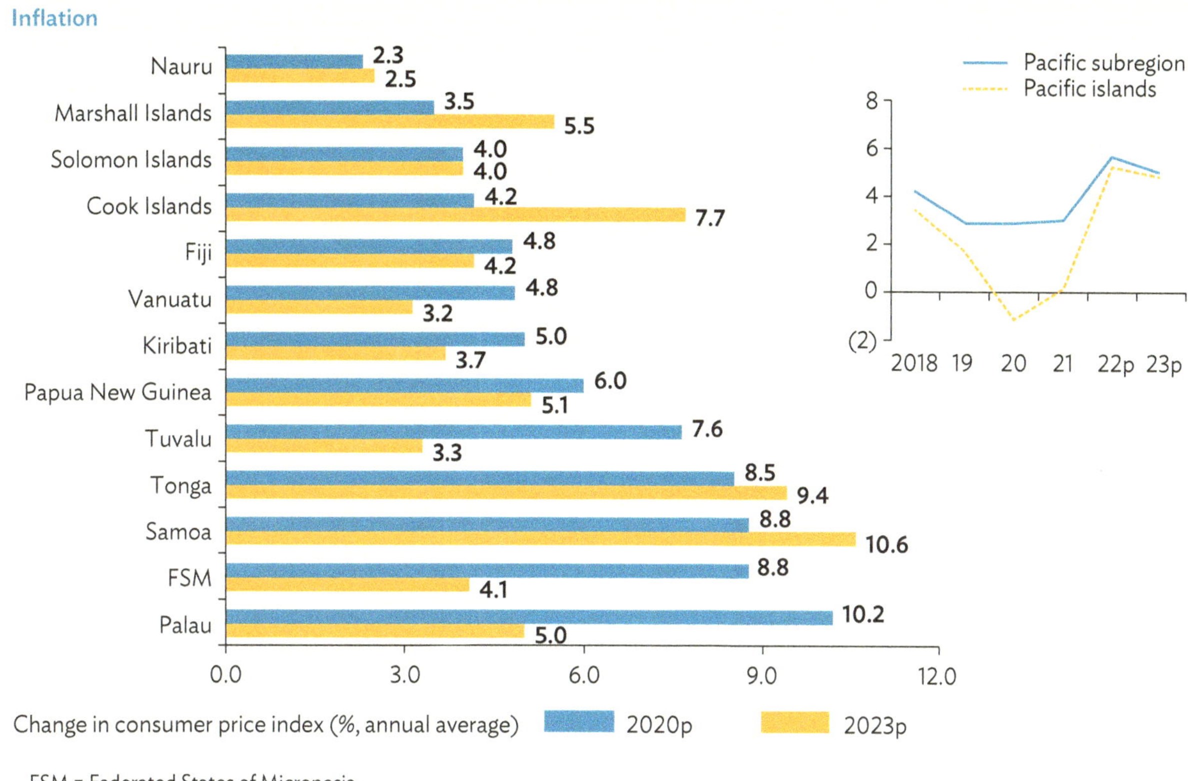

Figure 3: Inflation in Pacific Countries, 2022 and 2023

FSM = Federated States of Micronesia.
Source: *ADB Pacific Economic Monitor*. December 2022.

more severely, as they spend a larger proportion of their income on basic goods and services, whose prices are more sensitive to inflation. Given that women generally have lower incomes than men, they are more vulnerable to these inflationary pressures. This compounds the existing gender disparities in economic outcomes.

The pandemic stimulus and expenditures, combined with contractions in revenue, have led to increased public debt in Pacific island countries. This will likely result in reduced government expenditures, which may impact women and highly gendered expenditure, for example, social spending. Levels of debt varied considerably among Pacific island countries before the COVID-19 pandemic, averaging just over 32% of GDP in 2019, (but ranging from 62% of GDP in Nauru to 8.2% in Solomon Islands).[44] The average debt-to-GDP ratio in the region after COVID-19 was 40% of GDP, almost a 10-percentage point increase from 2019 (footnote 44). Most of the debt incurred was due to support stimulus funding during this period and was financed by multilateral development banks including ADB, the World Bank, and the International Monetary Fund, under concessional terms (footnote 44). Debt was particularly significant in tourism-reliant economies and commodity-exporting countries, which saw their fiscal positions worsen because of falling

---

[44]   S. Roger. 2022. *Debt Landscape and Fiscal Management Issues in Pacific Small Island Developing States*. Background paper provided at the Pacific Regional Debt Conference, online, 5–8 April.

commodity prices. Several countries in the region are at high risk of debt distress and have a limited ability to withstand further economic shocks (footnote 42). This reduced fiscal capacity and debt servicing burdens will likely impact other key investments. For example, the fiscal costs of future disasters triggered by natural hazards may exceed the historical average of 1.1%–1.5% of GDP per year, requiring more government surplus, not less.[45] Decreased government expenditures are likely to have a disproportionate impact on those sectors impacting women.

More broadly, there is an opportunity to look at the impact and prioritization of gender-focused development assistance in the region. Research shows that in the Pacific, gender-focused official development assistance from Australia, the largest bilateral donor in the region, tends to focus on countries where women's empowerment is higher, as represented by political representation.[46] This has a paradoxical impact in that it is likely to be more effective but is not getting targeted to those women who likely need it the most (footnote 42).

---

[45]   H. Nishizawa, S. Roger, and H. Zhang. 2019. *Fiscal Buffers for Natural Disasters in Pacific Island Countries*. Quoted in S. Roger. 2022, *Debt Landscape and Fiscal Management Issues in Pacific Small Island Developing States*. Background paper provided at the Pacific Regional Debt Conference, online, 5–8 April.

[46]   Development Policy Centre and T. Wood. 2023. What is Australian Gender Equality Aid Spent on? What Brings Better Outcomes for Women? *Development Policy Centre Discussion Paper* No. 106.

VOICE, AGENCY, AND DECISION-MAKING DURING THE PANDEMIC

Several Pacific governments crafted COVID-19 national preparedness and response strategies with minimal input from women. Throughout the COVID-19 pandemic, women were inadequately represented in official leadership positions across the Pacific, with their political involvement recorded at 8.8% in 2020.[47] Studies have shown that the effectiveness of COVID-19 health responses were largely political in nature.[48] The minimal participation of women in leadership and decision-making roles, coupled with the absence of women's ministries from COVID-19 task forces in many instances, resulted in women and vulnerable groups being insufficiently consulted or represented during most COVID-19 response planning efforts (footnote 49). Only 23% of women leaders were aware of consultation processes with women's organizations for COVID-19 response plans (Figure 4).[49]

Has the government consulted women's organizations in COVID-19 response efforts?

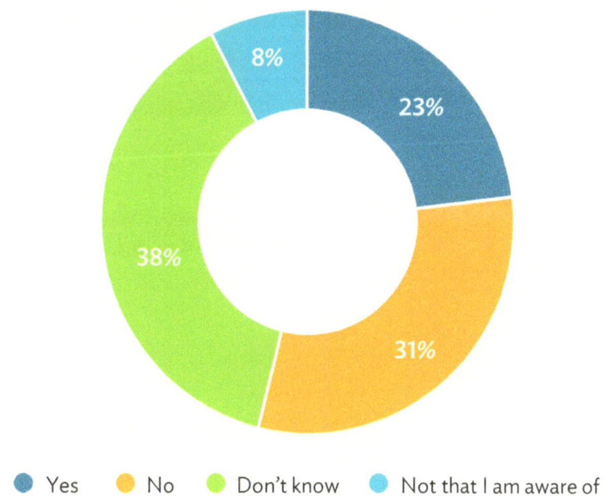

COVID-19 = coronavirus disease.
Source: Shifting the Power Coalition. 2020. *Mobilising Women's Leadership: Solutions for Protection and Recovery in a time of COVID-19 and TC Harold.*

---

47   Pacific Women in Politics. 2022. *National Women MPs*.

48   G. Phillips et al. 2022. Lessons from the Frontline: Leadership and Governance Experiences in the COVID-19 Pandemic Response across the Pacific Region. *The Lancet Regional Health: Western Pacific*. 5.100518.

49   Shifting the Power Coalition. 2020. *Mobilising Women's Leadership: Solutions for Protection and Recovery in a time of COVID-19 and TC Harold.*

Government COVID-19 response and recovery plans often did not mainstream gender analysis and initiatives across all strategic areas. As an example, Vanuatu's Tumi Evriwan Tugeta Recovery Strategy 2020–2023 for Tropical Cyclone Harold and COVID-19 did not include any explicit goals or plans to tackle GBV or enhance women's economic empowerment.[50] The Fiji Coronavirus Preparedness and Response Plan included no gender analysis or specific actions for women and girls.[51] The Tongan Ministry of Health COVID-19 Preparedness and Response Plan included limited actions on gender, but listed pregnant women as a specific cohort in measures focused on treatment for infection.[52]

Women were underrepresented in national health leadership and decision-making about COVID-19 prevention and control measures. Gender-disaggregated data on membership were not available for all COVID-19 task forces in Pacific island countries. However, where information was available, namely Fiji's COVID-19 Risk Mitigation Task Force and PNG's Ministerial Committee on Coronavirus, there were no female members in either task force.[53] Information on the full gender composition of membership for other Pacific island country COVID-19 task forces was unavailable. In some cases, information on leadership is available, showing only two female-led task forces: the Cook Islands Health Emergency Task Force and the Fiji COVID-19 Vaccine Task Force. Fiji also had a stand-alone COVID-19 Response Gender Working Group, led by the Ministry of Women, Children, and Poverty Alleviation (footnote 18).

Women were less likely to be in positions to influence or create infection prevention and control policies. In the Pacific region, nurses comprised more than 74% of the health workforce, yet despite this, there was little evidence of nurses having a concomitant influence on hospital policy and regulation.[54] An analysis of the global influence of nurses on health policy revealed that hierarchical structures in health care, gender-based power dynamics, and insufficient confidence and skills collectively hindered nurses' ability to contribute significantly to policies, including those directly relevant to nursing.[55] Despite this, researchers found that the patriarchal structure of Pacific societies ensured male voices were heard and male leadership was magnified, even if women health care workers had more experience or provided most of the health care service.[56]

Where women were in health leadership positions, research shows that they demonstrated a strong, inclusive leadership style that "empowered and united their colleagues to feel confident and work together in navigating the workplace unease and pressures ushered in by the COVID-19 pandemic" (footnote 56).

---

[50]   Government of Vanuatu. 2020. *Vanuatu Recovery Strategy 2020-2023: TC Harold and COVID-19*.

[51]   Ministry of Health and Medical Services Fiji. 2020. *Fiji Coronavirus Preparedness and Response Plan*.

[52]   Ministry of Health Tonga. 2020. *Ministry of Health COVID-19 Preparedness and Response Plan*.

[53]   UNDP. *COVID-19 Global Gender Response Tracker* (accessed 22 March 2022).

[54]   M. Rumsey, et al. 2022. Achieving Universal Health Care in the Pacific: The Need for Nursing and Midwifery Leadership. *The Lancet Regional Health: Western Pacific*. 19. 100340.

[55]   S. P. Rasheed, A. Younas, and F. Mehdi. 2020. Challenges, Extent of Involvement, and the Impact of Nurses' Involvement in Politics and Policy Making in in Last Two Decades: An Integrative Review. *Journal of Nursing Scholarship*. 52(4), pp. 446–455.

[56]   G. Phillips, et al. 2023. Women on the Frontline: Exploring the Gendered Experience for Pacific Healthcare Workers during the COVID-19 Pandemic. *The Lancet*. 42. 100961.

The marginalization of women and girls' voices was mirrored at both community and household levels during the COVID-19 crisis. Preexisting patterns of household decision-making persisted in decisions related to COVID-19 preparation and response. A study in Solomon Islands highlighted that when asked who was primarily responsible for making decisions for their households regarding COVID-19 readiness, most respondents identified men. Similarly, decisions regarding community-level preparedness and response were predominantly attributed to chiefs, elders, church leaders, and members of community committees, with few mentioning women's leaders (3 out of 80 interviewees) or youth leaders (two mentioned).

WOMEN AND HEALTH

Access to Vaccines

The Pacific governments' ability to deliver gender-responsive COVID-19 measures was hindered by the limited collection of sex-disaggregated data across all countries capturing COVID-19 case numbers, hospitalizations, vaccination, and mortality rates.[57] While official data were not collected for most countries, mortality rates were captured by the Fiji Ministry of Health and Medical Services, with data disaggregated by gender, age, location, and vaccination status.[58] It recorded a cumulative total of 1,298 COVID-19-related deaths, with 54.6% (380) occurring among males and four deaths classified as maternal deaths (footnote 58).

In the initial stages of the vaccine rollout, women were less likely to receive a COVID-19 vaccine in several Pacific island countries. Government data from PNG showed a gender variance in vaccination rates. PNG reported one of the lowest vaccination rates globally, with only 3.6% of the population having received at least one dose, and men being twice as likely as women to have received a dose.[59] A study conducted in Kiribati, PNG, Samoa, Solomon Islands, and Tonga found that women were less likely than men to have received the first two doses of a COVID-19 vaccine (footnote 14). The study found that this was particularly true among older women and those residing in urban areas. The most frequently noted reason for not completing their full course was availability-related: for example, individuals waiting for their scheduled second dose, coupled with concerns about potential side effects (footnote 14). The study also found some women were also concerned about the overall effects on reproductive health (Figure 5).[60]

Practical obstacles affected the vaccination uptake among women in Fiji. A survey by the Fiji Women's Rights Movement found that 58% of women stated nothing would stop them from having the COVID-19 vaccine, 13.5% identified transport and distance as barriers to vaccination, and 9.8% saw registering online with required documents as a key.[61]

---

57 Databases reviewed: World Health Organization. *COVID-19 Dashboard*; United Nations Children's Fund (UNICEF). *COVerAGE Database*, GLOBAL Health 5050. *The COVID-19 Sex-Disaggregated Data Tracker*; and UN Women. *COVID-19 and Gender Monitor* (accessed 15 August 2024).

58 N. Sharma et al. 2022. Descriptive Analysis of Deaths Associated with COVID-19 in Fiji, 15 April to 14 November. *Western Pacific Surveillance and Response*. 13(4).

59 GLOBAL Health 5050. *The COVID-19 Sex-Disaggregated Data Tracker* (accessed 15 August 2024).

60 The results for Samoa in this survey contradict data published by the Ministry of Health in Samoa in February 2022 showing more women have received two doses of the COVID-19 vaccine than men. This may be a result of the vaccine rollout being at a different stage at the time the survey was conducted.

61 Fiji Women's Rights Movement. 2021. *Rapid Assessment: Fijian Women's Perceptions of the COVID-19 Vaccine*.

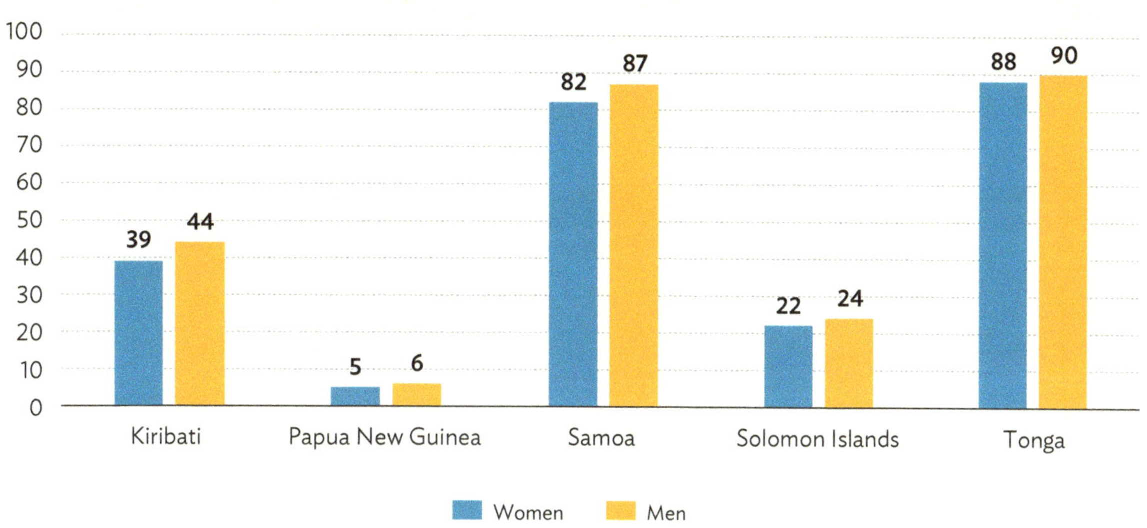

Source: Asian Development Bank and UN Women. 2022. *Two Years On: The Lingering Gender Effects of COVID-19 in Asia and the Pacific.*

Barriers to Accessing Health Systems

The pandemic placed further strain on fragile health systems and disrupted the delivery of essential services. The pandemic impacted the accessibility and availability of health care services, including sexual and reproductive health (SRH) services for women and girls (footnote 10). While certain services continued operating under normal conditions, others were limited by reduced capacity, shortened operating hours, or revised referral protocols. Referrals sometimes directed individuals to services located farther away, posing particular difficulties for women and girls, especially if these facilities were situated in unsafe areas or faced travel restrictions imposed by their families. Challenges such as transport disruptions, movement limitations, concerns about contracting the virus, unfamiliarity with new procedures and operational hours, and compromised confidentiality due to movement restrictions were identified as additional barriers to accessing health care. Interviewees also noted shortages of medications and reduced staffing levels at health centers.[62] There were also limitations in accessing SRH services due to infection prevention protocols to limit large-scale community transmissions.

[62]   Tonga Statistics Department. 2018. *Tonga Labour Force Survey 2018*; Pacific Community and Tuvalu Central Statistics Division. 2018. Tuvalu HIES Report 2015-2016: Full Report. Noumea, New Caledonia: Pacific Community (SPC). Quoted in International Labour Organization. ILOSTAT Database (accessed 25 March 2022).

Women Health Care Workers

As shown in Figure 6, women comprised the majority of the health care workforce in Pacific island countries, in particular, the nursing and midwifery workforce. In Tonga and Tuvalu, over 80% of health care staff were women (footnote 62). While women comprised a substantial portion of the health care workforce and were disproportionately represented in roles with high volume patient contact. Analysis of the COVID-19 impact on women in the Pacific indicates that they often provided emotional and spiritual support to patients, alongside their medical responsibilities and were often at the forefront of exposure and risk during the pandemic response (footnote 56).

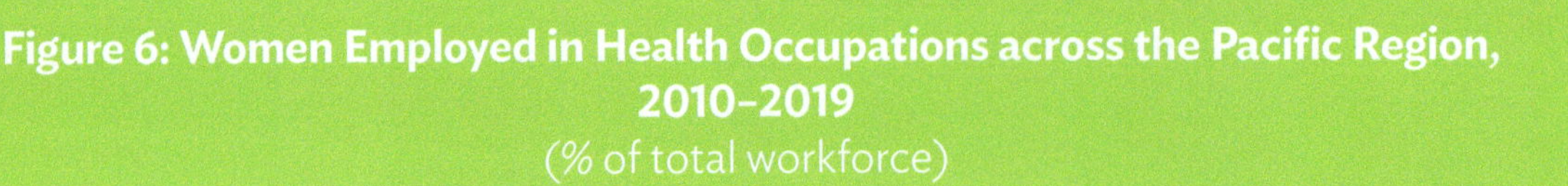

Figure 6: Women Employed in Health Occupations across the Pacific Region, 2010–2019
(% of total workforce)

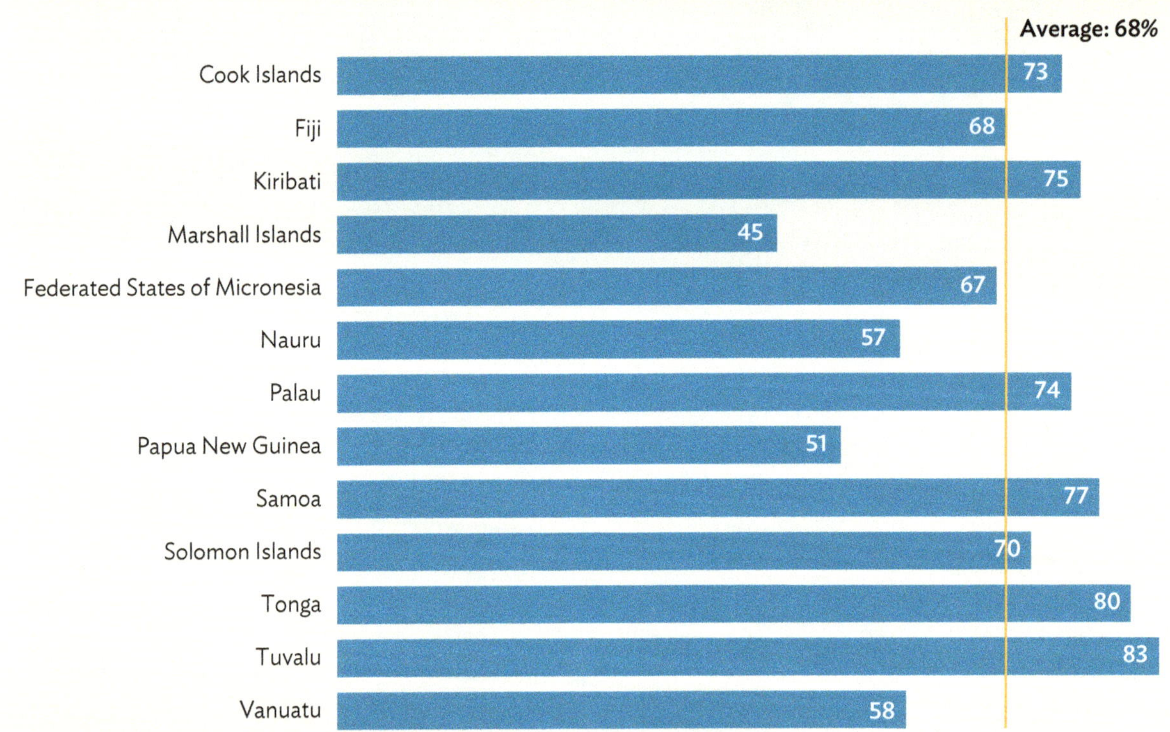

Source: International Labour Organization. *ILOSTAT Database* (accessed 13 August 2024).

Disruptions in Access to Critical Women's Health Services, Including Sexual and Reproductive Health and Rights

The pandemic highlighted and potentially worsened existing gaps in health care, notably the diagnostic gap where women and girls are often underdiagnosed or diagnosed late for conditions such as diabetes and cancer. This discrepancy in diagnosis and treatment was likely intensified as health care resources were reallocated and routine services became less accessible during the pandemic. The COVID-19 pandemic disrupted essential health services worldwide for more than 2 years, resulting in interruptions to routine childhood immunizations, including in Fiji.[63] The break in the vaccination schedule left many children without crucial protection against diseases like measles.

Due to COVID-19, fewer children were able to access primary health care services. There are predictions, but no current data, regarding reduced rates of childhood vaccination due to service limitations in response to the pandemic.[64] The United Nations Children's Fund (UNICEF) estimated that "thousands" of children in the Pacific are at risk of missing vaccinations due to COVID-19 measures, despite increased vaccine awareness in the region following the 2019 Pacific measles outbreak.[65] Global evidence does show some decline in childhood vaccination rates due to barriers in health care access.[66] Learnings from previous epidemics have shown the knock-on effect of barriers to health care and declining rates of childhood vaccination, with women taking time off work to care for their sick children.[67]

Access to SRH services for women and girls was disrupted in certain areas, compromising their rights in some cases. In some locations, midwives and nurses were redeployed for COVID-19 preparedness and response, reducing the ability of these professionals to deliver clinical SRH services. Disruptions in transportation, travel restrictions, and shortages of supplies contributed to decreased access to contraception and limited information about SRH services.[68]

Lockdown measures affected the production and supply chains of contraceptives, leading to reports that several major manufacturers in Asia reduced their operational capacity.[69] Travel restrictions and rationing of both air and sea freight within the Pacific region severely limited the supply chain for all imported goods, including for essential medicines, PPE, and vaccines. There was also evidence that gaps in forecasting and procurement of supplies led to low supplies and stock-outs.[70]

---

[63]　S. Sharma. 2022. *Protecting the Most At-Risk Children | UNICEF Pacific Islands*. 16 December.

[64]　Gender in Humanitarian Action and Gender-Based Violence Area of Responsibility. 2021. *Gender and COVID-19 Vaccines: Listening to Women-Focused Organizations in Asia and the Pacific*.

[65]　UNICEF. 2020. *As COVID-19 Threatens, Pacific Children's Lives Are at Stake with Many Children at Risk of Missing Out On Basic Vaccines*. Press release, 27 April.

[66]　WHO. 2021. *COVID-19 Pandemic Leads to Major Backsliding on Childhood Vaccinations, New WHO, UNICEF Data Shows*. 15 July.

[67]　H. Simba and S. Ngocobo. 2020. *Are Pandemics Gender Neutral? Women's Health and COVID-19*. Frontiers in Global Women's Health.

[68]　Specialist Health Services. 2020. *Mid Term Review: Transformative Agenda for Women, Adolescents and Youth in the Pacific: Towards Zero Unmet Need for Family Planning Strategic input on health to the Australian Government*.

[69]　C. Purdy. 2020. *How Will COVID-19 Affect Global Access To Contraceptives – And What Can We Do About It?* Devex. 11 March.

[70]　A. Dawson et al. 2021. *The COVID-19 Pandemic and Sexual and Reproductive Health Rights in the Pacific*.

Child and maternal mortality rates across the Pacific were on the rise prior to the pandemic and challenges to balancing health service provision with pandemic response created additional barriers for women accessing care.[71] There were reports of pregnant women being turned away from facilities due to the providers' fear of exposure to COVID-19, and confusion regarding pre-triage procedures for emergency and routine care at hospitals (footnote 71). In PNG, the head of Obstetrics and Gynecology at the University of Papua New Guinea indicated that COVID-19 had heightened the risks associated with pregnancy for both women and their babies.[72]

Menstruation became more difficult to manage during the pandemic. Evidence from Fiji, PNG, and Solomon Islands shows that a scarcity of menstrual hygiene management products, a lack of water for washing, the impact of lockdowns, alongside the increased cost of using paid public toilets, and the closure of some toilets in public spaces exacerbated difficulties in menstruation management. Almost one-third (30%) of girls and women surveyed in the Pacific said that period products had become harder to find during the pandemic.[73]

Menstrual hygiene products in Fiji, PNG, and Solomon Islands increased in cost and there was a scarcity of some items. Women reported both complete stock-outs and having less choice in their preferred product and brand since the pandemic. There was some evidence that scarcity particularly impacted supplies in rural areas (footnote 73). According to a survey conducted in Fiji, PNG, Solomon Islands, and Vanuatu, 22% of women and girls noted that menstrual hygiene products had become more costly since the start of the pandemic, attributed to reduced income availability and disruptions in supply chains.[74] Women in Fiji observed price increases ranging from F$0.50 to F$3 per packet of menstrual hygiene products (footnote 74).

Access to COVID-19 Information and Prevention Measures

Women's access to information about COVID-19 and vaccinations was impacted by low literacy, limited internet access, and the closure of women's spaces. Before COVID-19, gender disparities in literacy, education, and technology made women less likely to access reliable information about COVID-19 vaccinations. Additionally, the lockdown measures limited the face-to-face informal networks that women relied on (footnote 64). In PNG, more than 50% of survey respondents expressed hesitancy or uncertainty about accepting COVID-19 vaccines. The primary reason cited was insufficient knowledge about the vaccine (footnote 14).

During the COVID-19 pandemic, representatives from women's organizations, crisis response groups, and disability advocacy organizations highlighted the lack of suitable information as a challenge (footnote 10). Unclear information regarding lockdown measures and the disease contributed to panic and a rapid return to provinces during the initial phase. Messaging was sometimes not appropriately contextualized or simplified.[75]

---

71   WHO. 2017. *New UN Report Highlights Child Mortality Rates for the Pacific*.

72   N. Whiting. 2020. *Coronavirus Fears Leave Pregnant PNG Women at Risk Despite Nation's Low Infection Rate*. ABC News. 25 June.

73   Plan International. 2020. *Periods in a Pandemic: Menstrual Hygiene Management in the Time of COVID-19*.

74   Talei Tora. 2020. *Food Over Sanitary Pads: Women in Fiji Struggling to Cope with Periods in the Pandemic*. *The Guardian (Suva)*. 10 June.

75   United Nations (UN) Population Fund and Women Enabled International. 2021. *The Impact of COVID-19 on Women and Girls with Disabilities: A Global Assessment and Case Studies on Sexual and Reproductive Health and Rights, Gender-Based Violence, and Related Rights*.

A lack of accessible and appropriate information about COVID-19 restrictions for women with disabilities caused confusion and prevented them from accessing critical services. A study by Women Enabled International and the Pacific Disability Forum revealed that deaf individuals in Fiji received information during the COVID-19 pandemic that they could not leave their homes. Two participants mentioned they were too fearful to seek hospital care for maternity needs. Another survey conducted by the Psychiatric Survivors Association indicated that 65% of homeless individuals with psychosocial disabilities in Suva were unaware of the virus (footnote 9). Interviewees with psychosocial disabilities also mentioned a lack of access to mental health services during the COVID-19 lockdown.[76]

Research on women's communication preferences and channels for accessing COVID-19 information was limited. One survey conducted by the Fiji Women's Rights Movement found that 74% of female respondents cited the Fiji Ministry of Health and Medical Services website as their source of information on COVID-19 (footnote 61). This was closely followed by social media platforms, at 73%. Print media stood at 56%, compared to radio (53.3%) and the Government of Fiji website (51.4%) that female respondents cited as sources of information regarding COVID-19 (footnote 61). Evidence from other outbreaks, such as the measles outbreak in Samoa and Tonga in 2019, has shown the importance of inclusive, women-led, early warning and disaster information systems to an effective health emergency response.[77]

For some women in PNG, Solomon Islands, and Vanuatu, a scarcity of water resources impacted infection prevention measures. The Vanuatu Young Women for Change raised concerns about water issues affecting the Teoma and Eton communities, where women struggled to access water. Many communities did not have access to running water or basic hygiene and sanitation, impacting their ability to undertake preventive measures, such as regular handwashing.[78] In Solomon Islands, limitations in infrastructure and resources were cited as major reasons affecting handwashing behavior. Some individuals mentioned they stopped washing their hands at critical times due to insufficient water supply, distant handwashing stations, or a shortage of containers to carry water (footnote 10). ADB and UN Women found that the most common reason for a lack of access to water during the COVID-19 pandemic was piped water only being available on certain days (footnote 14).

---

[76]   Adventist Development and Relief Agency (ADRA), CARE, and Save the Children. 2021. *Fiji Gender, Disability and Inclusion Analysis COVID-19, TC Yasa, TC Ana*.

[77]   UN Office for Disaster Risk Reduction and Action Aid. 2022. *Inclusive and Accessible Multi-Hazard Early-Warning Systems: Learning from Women-Led Early-Warning Systems in the Pacific*.

[78]   Shifting the Power Coalition. 2020. *Mobilising Women's Leadership: Solutions for Protection and Recovery in a Time of COVID-19 and TC Harold*.

IMPACTS OF COVID-19 ON GENDER-BASED VIOLENCE AND ACCESS TO SERVICES

Gender-Based Violence Incidence Rates and Help-Seeking during the Pandemic

Women's crisis centers and other GBV service providers reported an increase in GBV since the start of the pandemic. The Fiji Women's Crisis Centre (FWCC) noted that incidents of violence against women rose in frequency and severity during the pandemic. This increase was attributed to stress related to unemployment, social confinement, and women facing barriers in accessing the formal justice system. During the initial 3 weeks of April 2020, FWCC observed a surge in domestic violence cases in Fiji, escalating from 87 incidents reported in February 2020 to 527 in April 2020—equivalent to the total reported for the entire year of 2019. FWCC also noted an increase in the severity of incidents, including the use of weapons, such as knives (footnote 9). In June 2020, the Fiji Civil Society Organizations Alliance for COVID-19 Humanitarian Response reported a 200% increase in incidents of violence against women, according to reports from its member organizations.[79] In Tonga, the Women and Children's Crisis Centre documented a 54% rise in reported cases across their facilities during the initial 15-day lockdown period in early 2020.[80] According to a survey conducted by UNICEF in PNG, 45% of respondents indicated a rise in physical violence against women and children during the lockdown.[81]

Many countries in the region reported an increase in calls to GBV helpline services, including a 606% increase in call volume from February to April 2020 in Fiji. The minister for Women, Children, and Poverty Alleviation in Fiji stated that calls related to domestic violence to the national helpline increased from 87 in February to 527 in April 2020.[82] Nearly half of the reported cases were directly attributed to the COVID-19 pandemic, including factors like movement restrictions and economic pressures on families. Approximately three-quarters of female callers reported experiencing physical violence. FWCC noted that the rise included new instances of relationship violence and an escalation of existing violence in already troubled situations (footnote 80). The Domestic Violence Helpline in Samoa reported a 150% increase in calls to its service in the first 6 months of 2020.[83] There was an increase in calls in a particular period of the pandemic and it is difficult to track increases across the entire duration of the COVID-19 pandemic. Even if many women had access to a phone, it is reported that many felt too scared to use it.[84]

79   Food and Agriculture Organization. 2020. *National Agri-food Systems and COVID-19 in Fiji*.

80   UN Women. 2020. *Across the Pacific, Crisis Centres Respond to COVID-19 Amid Natural Disasters*. 10 June.

81   UNICEF. 2020. *Issue Brief: COVID-19 and Girls' Education in East Asia and the Pacific*.

82   Ministry of Women, Children and Poverty Alleviation – Fiji. 2020. *Joint Press Release Ministry of Women, Children and Poverty Alleviation, Fiji Women Crisis Centre, Medical Services Pacific, UN Women*. Facebook. 4 May.

83   UN Women. 2020. T*he First 100 Days of COVID-19 in Asia and the Pacific: A Gender Lens*.

84   SPC Counselling Subcommittee of the RWG. 2021. Discussion paper on domestic violence counselling to inform the RWG on the impact of COVID-19 and Tropical Cyclones Harold, Yasa, and Ana on gender-based violence/domestic violence counselling work in the region. Regional Working Group on Gender-Based Violence. 24–26 August.

Gender-Based Violence Services Availability and Accessibility

Some women did not feel safe at home and the COVID-19 pandemic cut them off from community support and important social settings that provided a safe space. Lockdowns, movement restrictions, and disruptions to programs and services resulted in reduced mobility and autonomy for women and girls. They were also isolated from their usual support systems and social networks, including colleagues, extended family members, and church groups (footnote 8). In PNG, a 2020 report stated: "Women are often at home with the perpetrator and with the lockdown. It also made it difficult to go elsewhere."[85]

Several countries in the region had limited or no formal safe shelter services for women and girls escaping violence prior to the COVID-19 pandemic, and some safe houses were closed or had limited capacity because of infection prevention and control measures. The limits on mobility and public safety concerns related to the pandemic impacted women's access to safe accommodation and likely caused some survivors to remain in their homes with their abuser. Safe houses in Kiribati, PNG, and Tonga experienced disruptions and closures to their services during the COVID-19 pandemic, while others had reduced capacity due to social distancing measures (footnote 12). Internal travel restrictions in Fiji, both on inter-island travel and to and from the two largest urban centers, Suva and Lautoka, reduced options for survivors seeking refuge.[86] In April 2020, the Christian Care Centre in Solomon Islands reduced its operations, admitting only high-risk clients (footnote 12). Many services returned to full capacity once initial lockdowns lifted and some services were able to adapt by offering hotel or guest house accommodation in lieu of space at the safe house. In some contexts, new services were opened during the pandemic. For example, in Kiribati, the closed safe house run by Our Lady of the Sacred Heart was replaced by a service run by the Kiribati Women and Children Support Centre (footnote 12). In Nauru, the dormant government-run safe house was refurbished and reopened through funding from the Australian Department of Foreign Affairs and Trade.[87]

In some countries in the region, there were barriers to accessing SRH services, with some clinicians redeployed for COVID-19. Despite this, there was no publicly available evidence about constraints either in the provision of or access to clinical management of rape services, nor is there information on any specific measures taken to ensure the continuity of access to these services.

The gender gap in internet access, which also existed for mobile phone ownership, made it impossible for some women to use digital or phone-based support services. The COVID-19 pandemic caused a broad shift in the delivery of GBV services remotely through telephone primarily, and in some cases, using chat or message functions.[88] The Pacific regional working group on the implementation of Family Protection legislation noted that some women did not have access to mobile phones to utilize the service, notably women from low-income households and those with hearing-related disabilities. They highlighted that even in contexts where survivors did have access to a mobile phone or the internet, they may have found accessing telephone counseling services difficult during COVID-19 lockdowns when they were confined at home and may have been closely monitored by the perpetrator.[89]

---

85   Monash Gender, Peace, and Security Centre. 2020. *Mapping the Impact of COVID-19 on Women, Peace and Security Practitioners in the Indo-Pacific Region*. Monash University.

86   Advancing Learning and Innovation on Gender Norms (ALIGN). 2020. *Action on COVID-19 and Gender: A Policy Review from Fiji*.

87   Government of Nauru. 2021. *WASDA 2020–2021 Annual Report*. Department of Women's and Social Development Affairs.

88   UN Women. 2020. *Early Preparations and Data-Gathering Mark Responses to COVID-19 in Fiji and Tonga*. 11 June; SPC. 2020. *Tonga Finding New Ways to Promote Human Rights for Vulnerable Women and Children*. 1 December.

89   SPC. 2021. *Proceedings of the 2nd Annual Meeting of The Regional Working Group on the Implementation of the Family Protection/Domestic Violence Legislation*.

Despite the constraints and documented impact of lockdown measures on service accessibility, there were efforts in many Pacific Island countries to strengthen GBV services and referral pathways in response to the COVID-19 pandemic (Figure 7). Many countries in the Northern Pacific opened GBV helplines or telephone counseling services for the first time, such as the FSM, Nauru, and the RMI.[90] Nauru refurbished and reopened the safe house, and in Tonga, the Women and Children's Crisis Centre expanded its services on outer islands, increasing outreach work, and opened a dedicated center in Vava'u.[91] The FSM, the RMI, and Vanuatu incorporated dedicated messaging on GBV into their broader COVID-19 awareness efforts. The FSM and Solomon Islands also revised their referral systems to enhance accessibility and incorporated additional health precautions related to COVID-19 (Figure 8).[92] Donors included support for GBV services in their COVID-19 support package, expanding existing investments to ensure continuity of services in the wake of increased demand.[93]

There were delays in and disruptions to access to justice for survivors in Fiji in the early stages of the COVID-19 pandemic. Cases of domestic violence faced delays in processing through the judiciary as a result of state of emergency measures. Additionally, strict enforcement of an overnight curfew led to more than 1,800 arrests within the initial 20 days of its implementation, causing further repercussions (footnote 86).

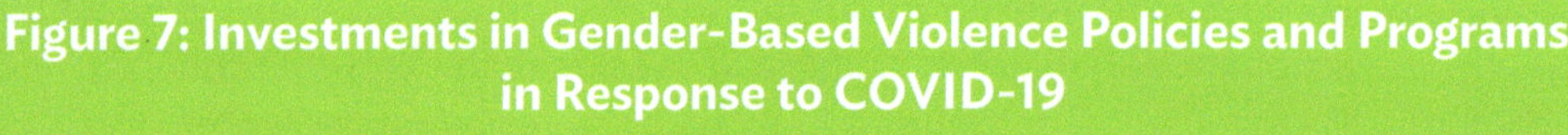

Figure 7: Investments in Gender-Based Violence Policies and Programs in Response to COVID-19

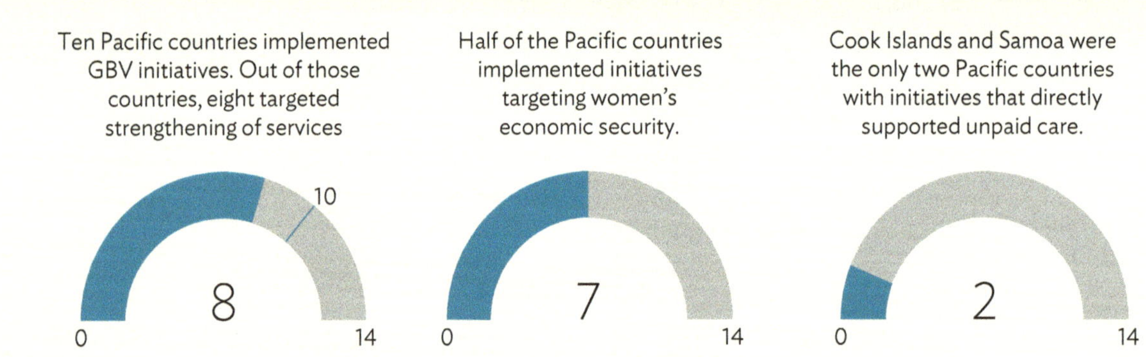

COVID-19 = coronavirus disease, GBV = gender-based violence.
Source: United Nations Development Programme. 2022. COVID-19 Global Gender Response Tracker.

90   Pacific Women Shaping Pacific Development. 2020. *Pilot Telephone Counselling Training for North Pacific Wraps Up*. 2 July.

91   Tongen Inepwineu Counseling Center. 2021. Review of Tonga Women and Children's Crisis Centre Outer Island Services.

92   SPC. 2020. *Submission to the Special Rapporteur on Violence against Women Office of the High Commissioner for Human Rights*.

93   Australian Department of Foreign Affairs and Trade. 2020. *Pacific Regional – COVID-19 Response Packages*; ADB. 2020. *Strengthening Gender Outcomes in Pacific COVID-19 Response and Recovery*.

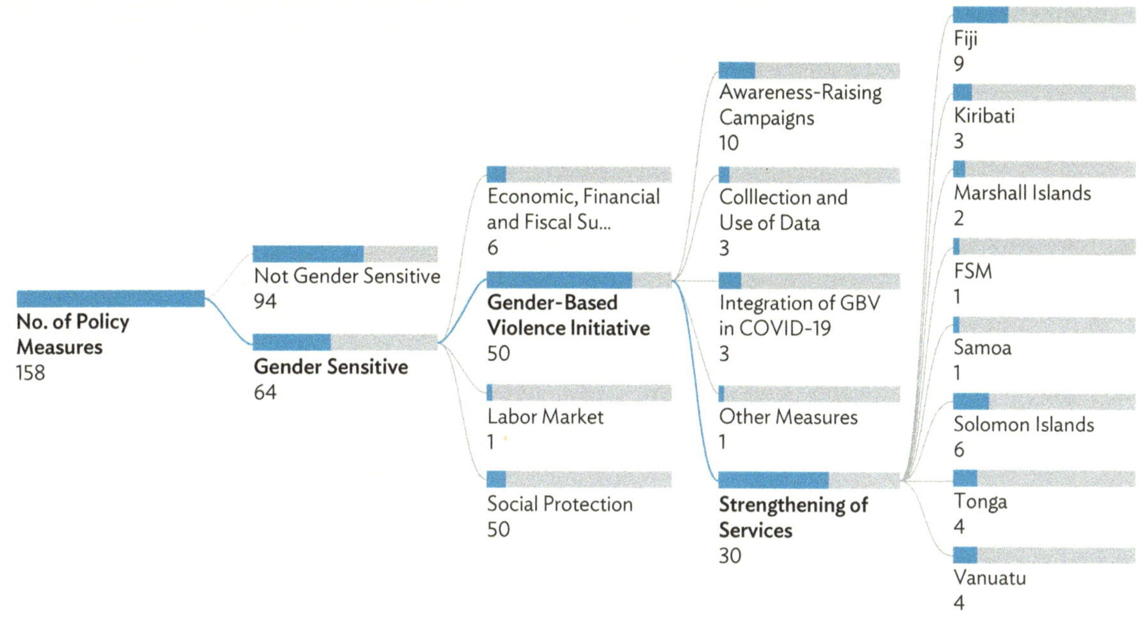

COVID-19 = coronavirus disease, FSM = Federated States of Micronesia, GBV = gender-based violence.
Source: United Nations Development Programme. 2022. COVID-19 Global Gender Response Tracker.

CHILD, EARLY, AND FORCED MARRIAGE, AND EARLY PREGNANCY

Although limited information is available, it shows the impact of the COVID-19 pandemic on CEFM (rates across the region despite some countries having high rates pre-pandemic). The combination of girls missing school and the economic impacts of the pandemic had the potential to increase rates of CEFM. The RMI (26%), Nauru (27%), and PNG (27%) had the highest rates of child marriage in the region, with rates likely to be even higher due to customary and informal cohabitation marriages that are often not officially registered.[94] A World Vision survey in PNG, Solomon Islands, Timor-Leste, and Vanuatu found 1.5% of households surveyed turned to early marriage as a coping mechanism in response to the economic shock caused by the COVID-19 pandemic.[95]

Quantitative data on the impact of the COVID-19 pandemic on rates of early pregnancy were not available, although some qualitative information pointed to an increase. Pre-pandemic data show that adolescent birth rates were rising in nine Pacific island countries.[96] Evidence from PNG suggested early pregnancy rates increased during school closures, while estimates from Fiji have suggested an increase in unwanted pregnancies because of the pandemic.[97]

---

[94] In PNG, the Marriage Act 1963 recognizes customary marriages. Under the traditional justice system, administered by village courts, readiness for marriage is determined by maturity, allowing girls to be married as soon as they start their period.

[95] World Vision. 2021. *Pacific Aftershocks: Unmasking the Impact of COVID-19 on Lives and Livelihoods in the Pacific and Timor-Leste*. Timor-Leste is not covered in this literature review: however, the data published by World Vision provide only an aggregate finding across all countries.

[96] UNFPA. 2020. *Editorial: The Pacific Can Become A Global Leader In Ending Child Marriage*.

[97] KORE Global. 2022. *The Impact of the COVID-19 Pandemic on Girls' Education and Wellbeing in Pacific Island Countries*. Australian Department of Foreign Affairs and Trade.

IMPACTS ON GIRLS' EDUCATION

There were moderate impacts on learning outcomes due to school closures (Figure 10), but information on gender differences is limited. Estimates for learners affected by school closures, throughout the region, show that slightly more boys than girls were impacted (Figure 9).[98] Findings on learning losses from PNG, Samoa, and Vanuatu showed mixed evidence, with disaggregated results data for Samoa and Vanuatu showing greater impacts for girls, although repetition rates were higher for boys in Samoa.[99]

Figure 9: Learners Affected by School Closures, Estimated, Male and Female

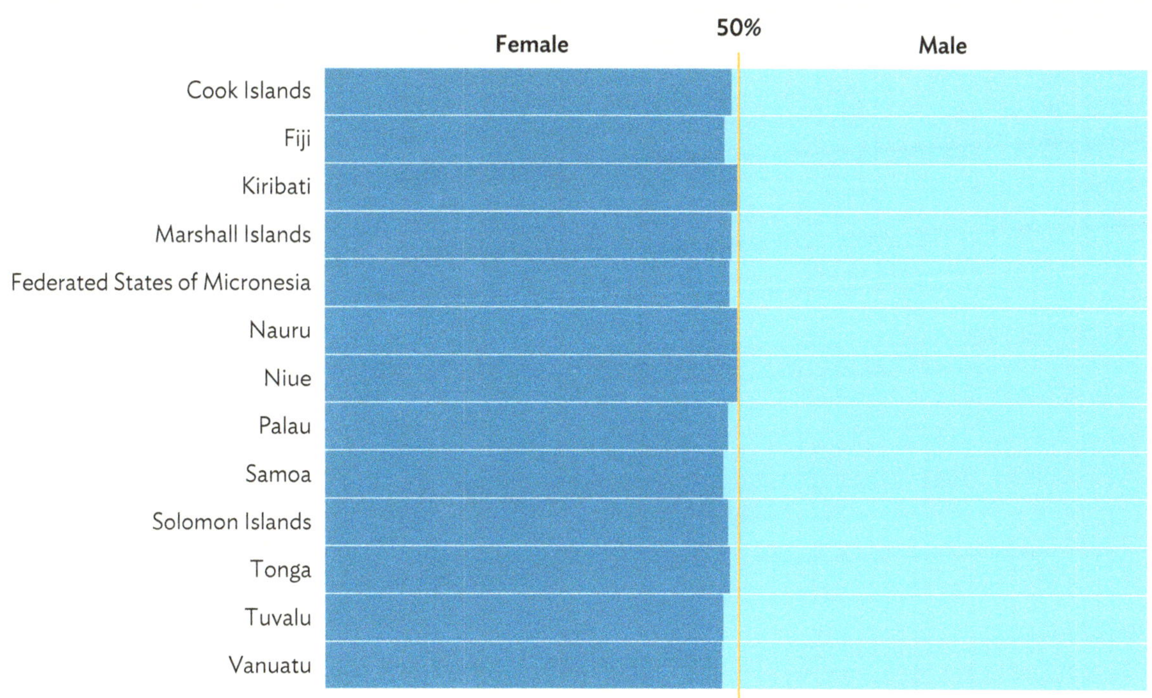

Note: Data are not available for Papua New Guinea.
Source: United Nations Educational, Scientific and Cultural Organization. UIS STAT Database (accessed 4 April 2022).

---

98   United Nations Educational, Scientific and Cultural Organization. *UIS STAT Database* (accessed 4 April 2022)

99   Plan International. 2021. *Smart, Successful, Strong: The Case for Investing in Adolescent Girls' Education In Aid and COVID-19 Response And Recovery*.

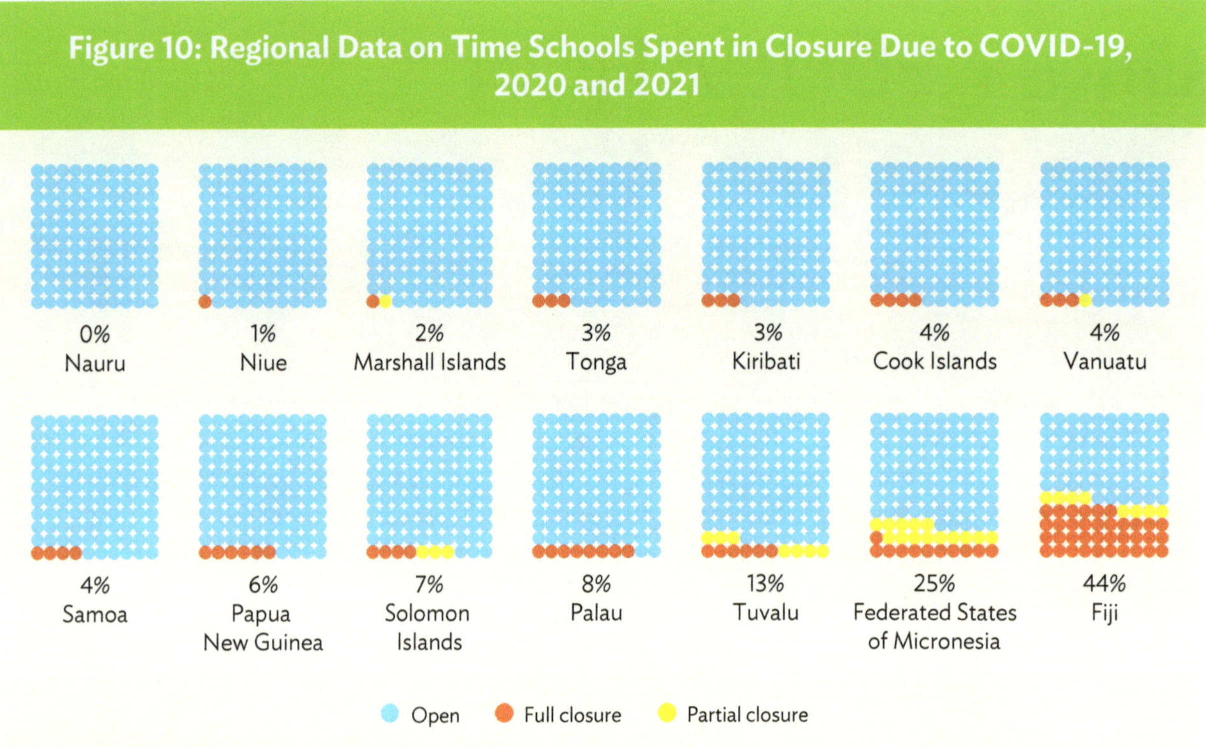

Figure 10: Regional Data on Time Schools Spent in Closure Due to COVID-19, 2020 and 2021

Source: United Nations Educational, Scientific and Cultural Organization. UIS STAT Database (accessed 4 April 2022).

Distance and online learning programs were not consistently available to girls, as only 38% of the region's population was estimated to have internet access.[100] A survey conducted by Pacific Women Shaping Pacific Development found that one in four girls surveyed could not do their schoolwork as they did not have internet access (footnote 16). This is corroborated by data from before the pandemic, indicating that mobile internet penetration in the Pacific is the lowest globally, with an estimated 38% of the region's population having access (footnote 100). There was also some evidence that specifically points to the risk of online violence and harassment as a barrier to home learning and online access for girls (footnote 99).

There were some data on retention and attendance at schools when they reopened; however, very little was sex-disaggregated. Information from surveys in PNG showed that, while most students returned to school, there was a delay in attendance among some. There was some indication that absenteeism was higher for girls than boys following schools reopening (footnote 97).

There was limited available information about the impact of the COVID-19 pandemic on affordability of education and any repercussions for girls' enrolment. Although primary education is free in all 14 Pacific island countries, several impose fees for junior or senior secondary education, which could pose affordability challenges for families experiencing reduced or lost income (footnote 8). A World Vision study conducted in PNG, Solomon Islands, and Vanuatu found that 14% of families resorted to sending their children to work as a coping mechanism for the economic impact of the COVID-19 pandemic (footnote 95).

---

100   Global System for Mobile Communications Association. 2019. *The Mobile Economy of Pacific Islands*.

RECOMMENDATIONS

Preparing for Disease X and Beyond

Preparing the Pacific communities, economies, and health systems for Disease X or future pandemics and health emergencies requires a gender-inclusive approach that learns from the COVID-19 pandemic. Addressing the specific needs of women, ensuring equitable access to resources and services, and integrating gender perspectives into health and economic policies are crucial steps in building resilient communities and health systems that can withstand future crises.

The COVID-19 pandemic disproportionately impacted women. The absence of sex-disaggregated data posed challenges in assessing the gender differences in the disease's spread and vaccination uptake, which is crucial for tailored health responses. Women experienced a surge in workload, a decrease in income and employment opportunities, and an increase in domestic violence, further diminishing their voice and opportunities.

Economic consequences were particularly severe in women-dominated sectors, as border closures led to a downturn in these areas. Women-owned businesses struggled with accessing finance and adapting services, exacerbating their economic vulnerability. Women were primarily responsible for managing the economic fallout, including ensuring food security and bearing the additional childcare burden during school closures. Lockdowns and mobility restrictions, intended as control measures, inadvertently led to a spike in domestic violence against women and girls.

The pandemic's impact extended to essential services, notably health care and education. The continuity, quality, and accessibility of these services were significantly disrupted, disproportionately affecting women and girls. This disruption manifested in delayed school returns for girls, limited access to online learning, and a reduction in the overall use of primary health care services by children. Furthermore, restrictions on maternal and child health services, along with sexual and reproductive health services, posed a risk to the progress made in reducing child and maternal mortality rates and in empowering women to control their fertility.

The pandemic's multifaceted impact on the Pacific region underscores the need for gender-sensitive approaches in addressing health crises and their broader socioeconomic effects.

Gender-Sensitive Surveillance and Early Warning Systems

Improve gender and disability disaggregated data and surveillance

Improving global disease surveillance and data systems is crucial for rapid access to information and swift response. This means investing in data collection methods that capture the experiences of all genders and those with disabilities, ensuring that their needs are not overlooked in crisis responses. Strengthening the detection and capacity of lab systems to do testing and monitoring will be critical, as will adopting a One Health approach.

A barrier to effective health system preparedness and management is a lack of gender- and disability-disaggregated data, as demonstrated during the COVID-19 pandemic. Without this data, it is challenging to understand how different groups are affected by health crises and to tailor responses accordingly.

1. *Integration and analysis of health data*

The integration and analysis of health data are crucial for better surveillance and response. This involves developing systems that can efficiently collect, integrate, and analyze data from diverse sources, providing a comprehensive picture of health trends and emerging threats. Such systems should be designed with a gender and disability lens.

2. *Gender-sensitive approaches to strengthening primary health care systems*

Strengthening primary health care is key to preparing for future health crises. Primary health care acts as the first point of contact for individuals, playing a crucial role in early detection and response to health issues. By investing in gender-sensitive primary health care, health systems can become more resilient, responsive, and inclusive. This involves ensuring that primary care facilities are accessible and equipped to meet the diverse needs of the population, including those related to gender and disability.

Promoting greater gender equality and supporting women's leadership in the health care sector are critical. As demonstrated in the COVID-19 pandemic, women were at the forefront of health care and represented the majority of health care workers. Greater efforts are needed to prepare systems to support work–family life balance, reduce burnout, offer mental health support, and offer greater recognition and leadership responsibilities that will better reflect the contribution of and support needed by the women's health care sector.

Gender-Inclusive Preparedness

Enhance consultation with women on preparedness and response plans

The lack of consultation with women and girls, and the limited number of women in key decision-making positions led to many instances of gender-blind COVID-19 response plans and policies. Continued and extended recovery planning and readiness should incorporate strategies focused on achieving gender equality and should be shaped by the specific needs of diverse women and girls, especially those from various backgrounds, such as single parents, women with disabilities, and those residing in rural areas.

Leverage artificial intelligence technology and technology for early detection and crisis management

The role of artificial intelligence (AI) and technology in health care is rapidly evolving. AI can aid in the early detection of health issues, predict outbreaks, and enhance crisis management. For instance, AI-driven data analysis can identify patterns indicating the emergence of a new disease, allowing for a swifter response. However, it is crucial to ensure that these technological solutions are accessible to all, including marginalized communities, and that they consider gender-specific health needs.

Ensure food security

Implement gender-inclusive strategies to mitigate the impact of pandemics on food supply chains, especially in regions heavily reliant on imported foods. Initiatives include supporting local food production. Special attention should be given to ensuring that women and girls, who are often responsible for household food preparation, have access to affordable and nutritious food options and safety nets.

Ensure inclusive and gender-informed public health measures

Ensure plans for quarantine, travel restrictions, and closure of public spaces are informed by some of the increased risks from evidence generated during the COVID-19 crisis, such as increased GBV. Incorporate explicit measures to address these risks. Public health campaigns to inform the public about the disease, its symptoms, and prevention methods are essential to reduce panic and misinformation. These campaigns need to be accessible to diverse groups of women, including those living in rural areas and those with disabilities.

Prepare accessible, inclusive, and secure health services and equipment

Ensure that gender is taken into consideration in the design of health care facilities, so that these are accessible and reduce risks, particularly in isolation units and intensive care facilities. It is essential to maintain reserves of vital medical supplies, including PPE, medications, and ventilators. This is particularly critical because shortages of PPE at the outset of the COVID-19 pandemic heightened risks for female health workers in the Pacific.

Develop plans for the continuity of essential services

The disruption of essential services, such as education and SRH services, had a dramatic impact on women during the COVID-19 pandemic. Ensuring uninterrupted access to health care, particularly SRH services, is crucial. This can be achieved by designating these services as essential and maintaining their operation during lockdowns, with contingent resources made available to the relevant implementing agencies. Telehealth services should be expanded to increase accessibility. Efforts must be made to reduce the stigma around SRH services and provide accurate information to counter misinformation, particularly concerning vaccinations and reproductive health.

Strengthen systems and collaboration

Governments, health care providers, community leaders, and international organizations must work in concert to develop resilient systems capable of responding to pandemics, environmental crises, and the proliferation of diseases. These collaborations should prioritize the unique needs of women, men, and people with disabilities, ensuring that responses are inclusive and equitable. For instance, during the COVID-19 pandemic, women—who served as primary caregivers—faced distinct challenges that required targeted support, such as access to childcare or mental health services. ADB and development partners should consider more effective strategies to keep gender equality at the forefront of crisis response, which was not always the case during the COVID-19 pandemic. Data and lessons learned from stimulus packages and other response mechanisms need to be examined, captured, and put in place.

Plan for vaccine equity and manufacturing and accessible supply chains

Equity in vaccine distribution and access is another key requirement for preparedness. It is essential to consider how vaccine distribution can be made accessible and equitable for all genders, including those in remote or marginalized communities.

Ensure gender-sensitive community involvement and public health education

Community preparedness and public health education are vital in managing health emergencies in the Pacific. Ensuring gender-sensitive community education about health risks, prevention methods, and response strategies can significantly enhance the overall preparedness of the health system. This education should be inclusive, considering the different ways in which health crises affect various genders and individuals with disabilities. Community leaders and organizations can play a key role in disseminating this information, ensuring it is accessible and relevant to all community members. Ensuring communication methods are accessible and in many different formats will be critical to overcoming the kinds of information constraints highlighted during the COVID-19 pandemic.

Response, Recovery, and Building Resilience

Improve social protection systems

The COVID-19 pandemic laid bare how some government support systems do not adequately meet the needs of women and people of diverse sexual orientation, gender identity, expression, and sex characteristics. Developing inclusive criteria and understanding the work and incomes of women can support improved social protection systems for recovery from the pandemic and into the future. This includes expanding coverage to reach women in informal sectors and vulnerable groups, such as single mothers, women with disabilities, and those in remote areas. Implementing direct cash transfers, food assistance, and unemployment benefits can provide immediate relief. Additionally, integrating a gender perspective in social protection policies ensures that the specific needs of women and girls are addressed, such as childcare support and protection against GBV.

Ensure stimulus benefits women and associated negative impacts are mitigated

The COVID-19 pandemic has underscored the need for economic stimulus packages that specifically address the needs of women. Women, particularly in the Pacific region, have been disproportionately affected by the economic downturn, with women-owned businesses experiencing greater revenue declines than those owned by men. It is crucial that stimulus packages effectively reach these women, especially those leading micro, small, and medium-sized enterprises. Stimulus measures need to include direct financial support, tax relief, and low-interest loans tailored for women-owned businesses. Additionally, it is vital to provide income support and subsidies that are responsive to women's needs.

Women often bear a disproportionate burden of unpaid care work and are overrepresented in low-wage sectors, making them more vulnerable to economic crises. Promoting access to insurance for disasters and economic shocks is critical for women, who face higher risks from these events. Affordable and accessible insurance schemes can offer much-needed financial security.

As countries aim to reduce their debt burden, they are encouraged to avoid cuts in public expenditure that would disproportionately impact women. It is also important to address the greater impact of inflation on women, who typically have lower incomes and spend more on basic necessities. Effective stimulus plans must mitigate these inflationary risks and prevent the exacerbation of gender inequalities.

Improve care infrastructure

Implement policies and plans to address the gender gap in unpaid household and care labor and its impact on the lives of women and girls. There is ample evidence showing the pandemic increased the already uneven divide in unpaid care work for women and girls in the region. There is a need to develop contextually appropriate whole-of-government approaches to reducing, redistributing, or renumerating care work. Measures to do this include the following:

(i) Support increased access to quality, affordable, and accessible early childhood care, education, and out-of-school-hours care as a key pillar of women's economic empowerment and equitable recovery from the impacts of pandemics. Early childhood development strategies are being discussed in regional forums such as the Pacific Early Childhood Development Forums, and some countries have begun adopting national policies.[101] Early childhood development provides an entry point for expanding high quality service provision to younger children and extending the hours to help working families. The support for expansion and strengthening of accessible childcare systems will require, in some countries, support for skills development of teachers and carers, service design, and accreditation systems. It will also require targeted communication to caregivers and accessible enrollment systems. Support must be built upon and fed into national-led systems and programs already in place.

(ii) Extend existing maternity leave provisions and legislate maternity and paternity leave for all. Access to maternity leave varies across the region, and many countries have only limited paid provisions and no paid paternity leave at all. In some instances, it is a public

---

101   ADB. 2023. *Women's Economic Empowerment in the Pacific Region: A Comprehensive Analysis of Existing Research and Data.*

sector policy, with no overarching legislation for the private sector.[102] Extending existing provisions and legislating maternity and paternity leave for all would support greater caregiving responsibilities for fathers.

(iii)   Support greater access to care services for older persons. Elder care is largely undertaken within family support networks and is often a gendered role as women are expected to take on the role of carer.[103] There is a need to expand on current policies and programs targeted toward the older population in the Pacific, to decrease the burden on informal women caregivers.

(iv)   Introduce programs and highlight role models that showcase men's role in caring and domestic labor. Evidence-based parenting programs that target greater inclusion of fathers in parenting and support positive parenting skills and peer support can be effective in redistributing some unpaid care labor.

Support gender-based violence services

Commit long-term funding to ensure the continuity of GBV services and the ability to respond to future health crises. Funding for GBV services throughout the region can be time-limited and donor-dependent (footnote 12). The pandemic led to a documented increase in support for GBV services in many Pacific island countries. Commitments to long-term funding are needed to ensure the continuity of these services and limit disruptions and closures of services, which are crucial for survivors and support trust and help-seeking behavior.

Strengthen women's economic resilience

Future pandemic responses should include targeted economic support for women-owned businesses and female entrepreneurs. This can involve providing accessible financial support, such as grants and low-interest loans, and implementing policies that support women-led enterprises, particularly in sectors most vulnerable to pandemic disruptions, such as tourism and handicrafts. Training and capacity-building programs in digital literacy and e-commerce should be provided to enable women to adapt to new market realities and sustain their businesses during lockdowns or travel restrictions.

Ensure targeted support to provide greater protection for future economic shocks such as training, social protection, insurance, access to finance, digitization of services, and improved infrastructure. It is critical that these measures reach those in the informal sector.

Addressing the digital divide will be a key enabler for women and girls throughout the region and help build resilience. Support to narrow the gender gap in internet access and mobile phone ownership would support women-owned businesses, women, and girls' access to lifesaving GBV services, online learning, and the facilitation of the delivery of appropriate and accessible health information and other services.

---

102   World Bank. 2023. *Women, Business and the Law. Parenthood.*

103   Australian Broadcasting Corporation. 2022. *How is Elderly Care Changing in the Pacific?* 27 July.

GLOSSARY

Term	Definition
Agency	Ability to use endowments (such as education, skills, and others) and take advantage of economic opportunities to achieve desired outcomes.
Child, early, and forced marriage	While there are variations between countries on the legal age to marry, it is generally accepted that child marriage occurs when one or both spouses are married before the age of 18. This encompasses both consensual and forced unions.[1]
Economic violence	Economic violence "involves making or attempting to make a person financially dependent by maintaining total control over financial resources, withholding access to money, and/or forbidding attendance at school or employment".[2]
Gender	"Gender refers to the roles, behaviors, activities, and attributes that a given society at a given time considers appropriate for men and women. In addition to the social attributes and opportunities associated with being male and female and the relationships between women and men, and girls and boys, gender also refers to the relations between women and men. These attributes, opportunities, and relationships are socially constructed and are learned through socialization processes. They are context- and/or time-specific and changeable. Gender determines what is expected, allowed, and valued in a woman or a man in a given context. In most societies, there are differences and inequalities between women and men in responsibilities assigned, activities undertaken, access to and control over resources, as well as decision-making opportunities. Gender is part of the broader sociocultural context, as are other important criteria for sociocultural analysis, including class, race, poverty level, ethnic group, sexual orientation, age, and others."[3]

---

1   United Nations Population Fund (UNFPA). 2022. *Child Marriage - Frequently Asked Questions*.

2   UN Women. 2023. *FAQs: Types of Violence against Women and Girls*.

3   UN Women. 2023. *Gender Mainstreaming Concepts and Definitions*.

Term	Definition
Gender-based violence	"Gender-based violence is an umbrella term for any harmful act that is perpetrated against a person's will, and that is based on socially ascribed (i.e., gender) differences between males and females. It includes acts that inflict physical, sexual, or mental harm or suffering, threats of such acts, coercion, and other deprivations of liberty. These acts can occur in public or in private."[4]
Informal economy	All economic activities by workers on economic units (for example, households, enterprises, or firms) that are—in law or practice—not covered by formal arrangements.[5] Formal arrangements entail work that provides legal or social protection.
Intersectionality	Intersectionality is the understanding that people experience varying degrees of disadvantage based on gender, race, religion, ethnicity, disability, age, indigeneity, and other characteristics. Women are not a homogenous group, and intersectionality acknowledges the different ways that people experience discrimination.
Sexual and reproductive health and rights	Sexual and reproductive health is a state of physical, emotional, mental, and social well-being in relation to all aspects of sexuality and reproduction, not merely the absence of disease, dysfunction, or infirmity.[6] Women's sexual and reproductive health is related to multiple human rights, including the right to life, the right to be free from torture, the right to health, the right to privacy, the right to education, and the prohibition of discrimination.[7]
Women-owned business	≥51% owned by a woman or women; or ≥20% owned by a woman or women; and have ≥1 woman as chief executive officer or chief operating officer (president or vice-president); and have ≥ 30% of the board of directors comprised of women, where a board exists (International Finance Corporation. IFC's Definitions of Targeted Sectors); and for those women entrepreneurs with a loan from a financial institution, the loan size at origination would be between $5,000 to $1 million[8]
Women's economic empowerment	Women have the ability to succeed and advance economically, and the power to make and act on economic decisions to enhance their well-being and position in society.[9]

[4]   Inter-Agency Standing Committee. 2015. *Guidelines for Integrating Gender-Based Violence Interventions in Humanitarian Action*.

[5]   International Labour Organization. 2012. *Informal Economy and Atypical Forms of Employment*.

[6]   World Health Organization. 2024. *Sexual and Reproductive Health and Rights*.

[7]   UN Office of the High Commissioner on Human Rights. 2022. *Sexual and Reproductive Health and Rights*.

[8]   Women Entrepreneurs Finance Initiative. 2018. *Women Entrepreneurs Finance Initiative (We-Fi): Creating Finance and Markets for All*.

[9]   R. Calder, S. Rickard, and K. Kalsi. 2020. *Measurement of Women's Economic Empowerment. Work and Opportunities for Women Helpdesk Guidance No. 2*. London.

REFERENCES

Australian Department of Foreign Affairs and Trade. 2020. *Pacific Regional – COVID-19 Response Packages.* https://www.dfat.gov.au/publications/development/covid-19-response-package-design-framework#:~:text=The%20Pacific%20COVID%2D19%20Response,position%20the%20region%20for%20recovery.

Government of Fiji, Ministry of Health. 2021. *COVID-19 Situation Update.* https://www.health.gov.fj/covid-19-situation-update-23/.

S. Howes and H. Liu. 2022. The Pacific: Emerging from COVID, Slowly. *DevPolicy Blog.* October 19. https://devpolicy.org/the-pacific-emerging-from-covid-slowly-20221019/.

M. Johnston et al. 2020. *Mapping the Impact of COVID-19 on Gender in the Indo-Pacific Region II: Views of Women, Peace, and Security Practitioners.* Monash Gender, Peace, and Security Centre. Monash University. https://bridges.monash.edu/articles/report/Mapping_the_Impact_of_COVID-19_in_the_Indo-Pacific_Region_II_Women_peace_and_security_practitioner_views/12936206.

Monash Gender, Peace, and Security Centre. 2020. *Mapping the Impact of COVID-19 on Women, Peace, and Security Practitioners in the Indo-Pacific Region.* Monash University. https://www.monash.edu/__data/assets/pdf_file/0005/2209496/COVID19-and-WPS-Research-Brief_FINAL.pdf.

Pacific Women Shaping Pacific Development. 2020. *GBV Support Services Situational Report.* https://www.dfat.gov.au/publications/development/pacific-women-shaping-pacific-development-six-year-evaluation-report-and-management-response.

United Nations Educational, Scientific and Cultural Organization (UNESCO). 2022. *UIS STAT Database.* http://data.uis.unesco.org/ (accessed 4 April 2022).

UNFPA and Women Enabled. 2021. *The Impact of COVID-19 on Women and Girls with Disabilities: A Global Assessment and Case Studies on Sexual and Reproductive Health and Rights, Gender-Based Violence, and Related Rights.* https://www.unfpa.org/featured-publication/impact-covid-19-women-and-girls-disabilities.

World Bank and UNICEF. 2022. *Solomon Islands High Frequency Phone Survey on COVID-19: Results from Round Two - Data Collection: December 2020–January 2021, and April 2021.* World Bank. https://openknowledge.worldbank.org/handle/10986/37194.